Fibromyalgia

Enjoying Life Without the Pain and Fog of Fibromyalgia

(The Incredibly Simple Methods to Reduce Your Paid and Suffering)

Sandra Spencer

I0095458

Published By **Andrew Zen**

Sandra Spencer

Fibromyalgia: Enjoying Life Without the Pain and Fog of Fibromyalgia (The Incredibly Simple Methods to Reduce Your Paid and Suffering)

ISBN 978-1-998901-04-3

No part of this guidebook shall be reproduced in any form without permission in writing from the publisher except in the case of brief quotations embodied in critical articles or reviews.

Legal & Disclaimer

The information contained in this ebook is not designed to replace or take the place of any form of medicine or professional medical advice. The information in this ebook has been provided for educational & entertainment purposes only.

The information contained in this book has been compiled from sources deemed reliable, and it is accurate to the best of the Author's knowledge; however, the Author cannot guarantee its accuracy and validity and cannot be held liable for any errors or omissions. Changes are periodically made to this book. You must consult your doctor or get professional medical advice before using any of the suggested remedies, techniques, or information in this book.

Table Of Contents

Chapter 1: Fibromyalgia.

Fibromyalgia Syndrome, more commonly known by the name Fibromyalgia Syndrome or simply Fibromyalgia is a chronic illness that is characterized by widespread pain, severe tenderness, fatigue, sleep disturbances and psychological distress. The exact cause of Fibromyalgia is not yet known.

Latin terms myo (meaning muscles), fibro ("meaning fibrous tissue") and algia [meaning pain] were used to derive the name of a particular disease.

Fibromyalgia may be mistakenly referred to as arthritis-like symptoms. Fibromyalgia can be considered similar to arthritis, as it is a rheumatic condition. It causes pain and affects the soft tissues and joints. It also causes fatigue and pain that interferes with everyday activities.

Fibromyalgia is similar to arthritis in that it doesn't cause pain or swelling to the muscles, joints, or other nearby tissues. However, Fibromyalgia is sometimes associated with rheumatic illnesses such as Ankylosing

Syphalitis, Rheumatoid and Systemic Lupus Erythematosus.

Fibromyalgia Facts & Figures

According to National Fibromyalgia Association data, the prevalence is around 3-6%. An estimated 200 to 400million people suffer from this disorder, and there are 10 million affected in the United States.

Fibromyalgia occurs most frequently in people between 20 and 50. With increasing age, the frequency of this condition increases. American College of Rheumatology has stated that Fibromyalgia affects 8 percent of 80-year-olds and above.

Fibromyalgia occurs more frequently in women. The 7:1 ratio between male and female sufferers is 7; with 75-90% being made up of patients who are female. This is not the only way Fibromyalgia affects people.

Fibromyalgia may be inherited. This illness can also be diagnosed in the family if you have grandparents, parents, aunts, uncles, and other relatives who are affected.

Fibromyalgia patients are required to be admitted at least once every three year. Annually, it results in 5.5 Million ambulatory healthcare visits. The disease costs an average of $3400 to $3600 per year, but can go up as high as $6000.

Fibromyalgia can lead to patients missing 17 days per week of work. Patients who have the condition are less productive than people who use just 6 leaves. Because of this, Fibromyalgia-afflicted individuals suffer from a lower quality of life (4.8 out of 10) and loss of work output.

It is more common for patients to develop depression due to its bothersome symptoms than in healthy individuals (3.4 times higher). Fibromyalgia is responsible for about 23 deaths annually. Some of these are suicides. This adds an additional strain to Fibromyalgia fatalities, with the majority usually due to related injuries.

What Causes Fibromyalgia

Fibromyalgia still remains a mystery, even though it is well-known in the modern era. It is believed that there are some environmental triggers as well as bodily changes that can cause this debilitating syndrome.

* Anomalous Pain Perception

The most widespread theory regarding Fibromyalgia involves abnormal pain messaging. According to this theory, people who suffer from Fibromyalgia have a "different" way they perceive pain signals. These reactions are thought to have occurred due to chemical changes in Central Nervous System.

Because the CNS, which consists of the brain, nerves, and the spinal chord, delivers impulses through specialized cells around the body, it is not surprising. Fibromyalgia may be caused when the mechanisms of the system are altered.

* Neurotransmitter imbalances

Fibromyalgia also stems from chemical imbalance. Research has shown that Fibromyalgia patients have low levels of serotonin. Dopamine, cortisol or noradrenaline are also affected. Fibromyalgia may be caused by low levels these hormones.

They play an important part in the interpretations of pain stimuli.

These transmitters can also regulate bodily processes, such as sleep, mood, anxiety, stress response, behavior, and appetite. Fibromyalgia could also be caused by disturbances of routine activities (such sleep disturbances or trauma).

* Stress

Fibromyalgia happens more often after stress, physical or emotional. In most cases, Fibromyalgia is triggered by one of the following events.

Surgery

o Birth

o Injury

o Infection

o Relationships that are abusive or problematic

o The Death of a Loved One

* Sleep Disturbances

Fibromyalgia, as it has been said, can be caused when there are sleep disturbances.

Before Fibromyalgia was a diagnosis, symptoms of the disease were treated with sleep problems.

Now, however, it is clear that people who don't sleep well have more pain than those with disturbed sleep. Fibromyalgia can also be caused by insomnia.

* Genetics

Fibromyalgia develops just as other illnesses. Fibromyalgia may be triggered by certain triggers. You might be affected if you are related to someone with Fibromyalgia.

* See Related Conditions

Fibromyalgia could be more common in those who have Rheumatic conditions, which are disorders that affect the bones and muscles. Rheumatoid Arthritis can be accompanied by Osteoarthritis. Lupus, Lupus, Osteoarthritis and Ankylosing Syptylitis are some examples.

* Obesity

Obesity, which is now a common problem in society, is considered the greatest threat. Obesity is linked to Fibromyalgia.

Paul Mork and his colleagues discovered that Fibromyalgia has a higher incidence in women with body mass indices over 25 (overweight to obese). Their risk is 60% to 70% greater than for women of normal weight. Women who do not exercise regularly or have a daily exercise time of one hour are at higher risk.

Fibromyalgia - Prognosis

Fibromyalgia has a long-term condition. However it is still a chronic condition. The prognosis is good due to the recent advances in diagnosis. Recent studies have shown that symptoms are not changing over a long time. About 25% to 35% reported feeling less pain after using new approved medications.

Even though there is a lot of people who have better prognosis rates, it is the multidisciplinary team approach that produces the best outcomes. Fibromyalgia sufferers who are treated by a doctor as well as mental health and alternative therapies experts, tend to have the best chance of managing their debilitating symptoms.

Fibromyalgia in children is more common than in adults. Children also have good prognosis. Research has shown that juvenile Fibromyalgia symptoms tend to diminish in the first two years.

Fibromyalgia prognosis are generally optimistic. However, people with disabilities or life crisis often get a poor diagnosis. Poor outcomes are usually due to factors like depression, anxiety, sleep disturbances, inability or pain to work, and other factors like insomnia. Fibromyalgia may also cause you to abuse sleeping pills, illegal drugs, or alcohol.

Fibromyalgia Signs

Fibromyalgia has many symptoms and can be very different from one person. Here are some of these symptoms:

O Widespread Pain

They complain about widespread pain. This discomfort can occur in many parts of the body. However, it most often affects the neck or back.

Fibromyalgia pains are often constant. Sometimes the discomfort is lessened and sometimes it is more severe. The pain characteristic varies. This could be any combination of the following:

Mild ache

o Burning sensation

o Stabbing, sharp pain

O Extreme Sensitivity

Fibromyalgia sufferers can also experience extreme sensitivity. Extreme sensitivity is an extreme condition in which even the slightest touch can cause pain. Hyperalgesia can be described as this.

A simple accident like hitting your elbow or something similar can cause a longer-lasting painful sensation. This characteristic is known as allodynia.

Fibromyalgia is more than just sensitive to touch. It can also make it difficult to eat, drink, light and smoke. These sensitivities, although not affecting the person physically, can lead the sufferer to develop Fibromyalgia symptoms.

O Stiffness

Fibromyalgia patients also experience stiffness. Stiffness can become severe if you settle on one position for a long time (e.g. if it has been 4 hours since you last sat in an office chair).

Fibromyalgia causes stiffness. This condition causes tightness and pain in the muscles, which can then lead to stiffness throughout the body.

O Headaches

Patients with headaches are those who feel pain or stiffness in the neck, shoulders and head. They can be as severe or mild as Migraine-like. Sometimes headaches can be accompanied or worsened by nausea.

O Fatigue

Fibromyalgia causes fatigue and other symptoms. This can vary from mild to severe fatigue that is easy to overcome, to exhaustion that is comparable to the flu. Fibromyalgia sufferers often have difficulty functioning throughout the day as a result of this symptom.

O Paresthesia

Paresthesia, another symptom in Fibromyalgia is described by "pins and needles". It can be felt in your hands, arms or legs. While it doesn't cause any pain, people who feel it report feeling itchy.

O Poor Sleep Quality

Fibromyalgia patients may complain of poor sleep quality even if they had a good night's sleep the night before. This is because the disorder can hinder the ability to enjoy deep sleep. This stage of sleep can be crucial as it allows your body to repair itself.

O "FibroFog"

Fibromyalgia affects more than just the physical body. It can also disrupt one's psychological health. Fibro-Fog, a symptom that disrupts learning and thinking among many other processes, is also known as Fibromyalgia.

The following is a common sign of "Fibro Fog", which can be seen in patients:

o Difficulty learning something new

o Memory Problems

o Attention and concentration issues

o Confused or slowed Speech

O Depression

Fibromyalgia is known for its effects on the mind and body. It can lead to depression.

Fibromyalgia patients are likely to have low levels for certain hormones. This can lead eventually to depression. Fibromyalgia symptoms can be difficult to manage in some cases.

O Anxiety

Anxiety can be defined as anxiety that is caused by worry, fear, or uneasiness. Although anxiety is something everyone experiences, some people find it hard to let go of it. Anxiety may be present in many mental conditions. Fibromyalgia sufferers can also experience anxiety. It can also occur due to an imbalance of noradrenaline/serotonin.

O Dysmenorrhea

Common among women is dysmenorrhea. This refers to a painful period. Fibromyalgia has been diagnosed in large numbers as a symptom of Fibromyalgia.

Dysmenorrhea pain usually affects the lower abdominal, but it can also radiate towards the back and thighs. The symptoms range from mild to severe, but they are always present. It can last anywhere up to 12 hours.

O Restless Legs Syndrome

This is a neurological disorder that causes a strong need to move the legs, and sometimes the arms. Fibromyalgia patients can also have this condition, which is known as Willis Ekbom Disease.

Aside from a need to move, restless legs syndrome may also include involuntary movements of the limbs (also known as periodic leg movements).

O Irritable Bowel Syndrome

Irritable Bowel Syndrome is an individual condition. However, it can also be a symptom in Fibromyalgia patients. These individuals may experience symptoms such as stomach bloating or pain. The result is that they may become diarrhoeic or constipated.

Diagnosing Fibromyalgia

Fibromyalgia symptoms such as fatigue, pain and mood swings can all be common. They can be signs and symptoms of other conditions than Fibromyalgia. Worse still, symptoms can vary in intensity and duration. Fibromyalgia often gets diagnosed late due to these reasons. It can cause increased discomfort and delayed treatment.

If you have the symptoms mentioned above, your doctor will likely order the following tests: You might be asked to take the following diagnostic tests.

* Complete Blood Count

* Erythrocyte Sedimentation Rate

* Serum Cholesterol

* Serum Calcium

* Vitamin D Levels

* Thyroid Function Tests

* Tests of Kidney and Liver Function

After you have exhausted all possibilities, your doctor may diagnose Fibromyalgia according to the American College of Rheumatology. Fibromyalgia must present the following symptoms:

* Widespread pain in 4 quadrants of the body with a duration of at minimum 3 months.

* Feelings such as fatigue, difficulty thinking, and waking awake tired.

In the past doctors had to examine the 18 points. Pain in 11 of these points indicated Fibromyalgia. Since pain can be temporary, a patient might feel tender at one point and have another 11 the next day. The doctors weren't certain about which pressure points were to be checked. This diagnostic criteria has been dropped from the guidelines as of 2010, although some practitioners still use them.

Fibromyalgia may co-exist with other illnesses. Your doctor will confirm if you have had any of these symptoms.

* Headaches

* Stress or anxiety

* Jaw aches

* Irritable bowel syndrome

* Urinating is difficult

Due to the fact that Fibromyalgia may develop from genetic factors, the doctor will gather a complete family history.

Fibromyalgia is a difficult diagnosis for many doctors. Scientists have created what they believe to be a precise diagnostic exam for Fibromyalgia. This kit is called FM/a and it identifies Fibromyalgia based upon immune system markers. This exam is not usually covered under medical insurance, and costs $700 per unit.

Chapter 2: Fibromyalgia And Medications

Fibromyalgia may cause pain, fatigue, and disruptions to sleep. To treat these symptoms, patients are typically prescribed the following medications.

O Pain Relievers

Fibromyalgia has a common symptom: widespread pain. This is why most pain management treatments are geared towards pain management. Paracetamol, an available over-the–counter pain killer, may be enough to ease mild discomfort.

Paracetamol's effects can be resisted by some people. Codeine may be prescribed for those who are not able to tolerate Paracetamol. Codeine is often packaged with Paracetamol. Codeine works by blocking pain impulses reaching the brain.

Codeine should not last more than 3 days. If you still feel pain three days later, be sure to consult your doctor.

Tramadol Hydrochloride is another strong painkiller for Fibromyalgia. It works by altering pain sensation chemicals. It is available as 50mg capsules. This product is recommended for mild to severe pain.

Do not forget to take these precautions if you are being prescribed stronger painkillers (Codeine, Tramadol).

* Be cautious when taking this drug. You shouldn't drink or use heavy machinery.

* Before taking any medication, be sure to review the label and remind yourself.

* If you are not able to take these medicines together with another medicine, consult your doctor.

These medications can be addictive and are better for pain than others. Also, the effectiveness of these medications may decrease over time. In this case, it might be necessary to take increased doses.

These painkillers can cause fatigue and diarrhea. Be sure to consult your doctor before you discontinue using this medication. You might experience withdrawal symptoms if you stop abruptly.

O Antidepressants

Although depression is a sign that Fibromyalgia is present, antidepressants have been prescribed to treat the pain. Fibromyalgia can develop when there is a low level of neurotransmitters. These medications can also increase neurotransmitter levels and help with pain relief.

Antidepressants are prescribed to treat depression. You may also experience less fatigue and sleep problems.

Fibromyalgia may be treated using a variety antidepressants. They include:

o Serotonin Norepinephrine Inhibitors

SNRIs, which are prescribed to treat anxiety or depression, prove to be one of the most effective medications for Fibromyalgia. Duloxetine or Cymbalta and Milnacipran hydrochloride are just two of three FDA approved medications.

o Cymbalta

Cymbalta has been approved by FDA June 2008. It enhances the levels of norepinephrine, serotonin. These neurotransmitters improve mood and control pain.

This capsule should be consumed at 60 milligrams per daily, but the first week can be started with only 30 milligrams. Do not miss any doses.

Cymbalta is known to cause stomach upset. Take this medication with meals. Cymbalta therapy could lead to liver failure. Avoid abruptly stopping Cymbalta treatment, as this could lead to side effects like headaches and nausea.

o Savella

Savella was approved by the FDA in June 2009. It is a tablet that can be used for Fibromyalgia in adults. Savella appears to be able to decrease fatigue and pain, according several studies.

Daily, you should take two equal doses. The first day starts at 12.5mgs. The daily intake will rise to 100mg, or 50mg twice daily, over the next week. This is the recommended daily dose. Your physician may increase it to 200 mg.

Savella can also cause dizziness, nausea and hot flushes.

o Tricyclic Antidepressants

These drugs increase norepinephrine levels and serotonin. Fibromyalgia patients are recommended to take these drugs as they usually have low levels.

In addition to boosting brain chemicals Amitriptyline/Elavil and Nortriptyline/Pamelor can also increase the effects Endorphins. These are the body's natural painkillers. They also help to ease sore muscles.

They can be very effective, but they have side effects like dry eyes, dry mouth, dizziness, drowsiness or constipation.

O Anti-epileptics

Fibromyalgia is also treated by anti-epileptics. In fact, this category was the original FDA approved drug for Fibromyalgia.

Pregabalin/Lyrica is the first approved treatment for Fibromyalgia. These medications work by decreasing nerve signals. It can calm nerve cells that are hypersensitive and provide pain relief in as little a week.

Lyrica, which comes in capsules, is taken in two separate doses daily. Depending on the doctor's recommendation, the recommended dosage is between 150 and 350 mg.

Lyrica shouldn't be stopped abruptly like other Fibromyalgia medicines. This could cause stomach upset, sleep disturbances, or diarrhea.

O Neuroleptics

These drugs are also known under the name "anti-psychotics" and are prescribed for chronic pain relief. These drugs work in the same way as anti-depressants. They can ease the symptoms both of anxiety and depression that are common with Fibromyalgia. They also encourage sleep, which can cause insomnia in patients with widespread pain.

Quetiapine and other neuroleptics have been investigated in numerous researches. Research published in 2012 in Journal of Clinical Psychopharmacology shows that Quetiapine can improve sleep and mood by giving 50 to 300mg per day for 12 weeks.

Olanzapine is an anti-psychotic which can be used to treat Fibromyalgia. According to a

2006 study, it can also reduce pain in Fibromyalgia patients.

O Muscle Relaxants

Fibromyalgia sufferers are frequently affected by stiffness and spasms. Cyclobenzaprine can be prescribed by your doctor to relieve this condition. This drug is used to stop painful muscle contractions.

Relaxants do more than stop muscle spasms. They are also prescribed for pain relief, fatigue, and sleep management.

Chapter 3: Fibromyalgia Therapy

Experts disagree on the best way to treat Fibromyalgia. Although medication can help reduce symptoms, it cannot cure the disease. This is why professionals recommend mind and body therapies, such those listed below. These therapies have been shown to be effective when combined with multidisciplinary treatment.

O Cognitive Behavioral Therapy / CBT

CBT is most commonly used for mood disorders. However CBT can also be used to address pain issues. It is therefore being used as an additional treatment for the disorder.

CBT (Coaching and Therapy) is a goal-oriented method of psychotherapy. It is based on the idea that your thinking affects how you act. Both can play a major role in your feelings.

It works quickly and can affect changes in thought patterns and behavior. This form of talk therapy is often performed one-on-1. However, it is also possible to do with a small group.

CBT sessions are a way for your therapist and you to gain control over your illness. He can give you tips and tricks to help you get over Fibromyalgia.

CBT can help patients in as little 10-20 minutes. This is the best thing about it. Many studies have shown that CBT can reduce pain and improve sleep. It can also lower depressive episodes and increase your confidence.

Fibromyalgia sufferers from all ages can benefit from this treatment. However, it's more effective for children. This therapy is not meant to cure Fibromyalgia patients by itself. It can however be combined with other treatments, such as exercise, to help ease the symptoms.

O Guided Imagery

Guided imagery is a form o psychotherapy that can relieve Fibromyalgia symptoms. Menzies et.al conducted a 2006 study. Al, patients who used audiotaped-guided imagery reported lower levels anxiety and pain.

Your therapist will ask if you would like to use guided imagery. He might ask you for pleasant scenarios to relax you. For instance, he may ask you what a perfect day looks like at the ocean.

With the aid of audiotapes, guided imagery can be done by anyone.

Guided imagery works by distracting the mind. Guided imagery encourages the individual to stop thinking about the disorder. When he's more relaxed, his pain sensations will be significantly reduced.

O Physical Therapy

Physical therapy helps to heal, prevent, treat and manage injuries and diseases. Although physical therapy cannot treat Fibromyalgia in its entirety, it can ease pain. Experts agree this therapy can aid Fibromyalgia patients.

These are some of the techniques physical therapists can use to teach an afflicted individual:

- A proper posture, which can help muscle function better.

o Selfmanagement skills that can treat Fibromyalgia.

o Exercises that can reduce stiffness and pain.

o Relaxation exercise that can reduce muscle tension.

o Exercises to increase muscle flexibility.

o Other exercises that build strength and increase range of motion

Fibromyalgia can easily be managed with different forms of physical therapy. Hydrotherapy, also known as cold-packing or moist heat, is the most common.

Cold packs tighten blood vessels, decreasing inflammation. Moist heat, by contrast, dilates blood vessels to improve blood flow. Increased bloodflow means that nutrients and oxygen can be delivered to more parts of our bodies.

Hydrotherapy also eliminates harmful toxins. It also speeds up the healing processes.

Hydrotherapy isn't the only option for Fibromyalgia.

o Deep-tissue massage

o Transcutaneous electrical nerve stimulation

o Stretching

o Muscle strengthening exercises

o Pain relief exercise

Fibromyalgia Relief Options

Dr. Mark Pellegrino from Fibromyalgia Expert says that the key is a well-balanced treatment approach. Doctors recommend that doctors consider the following alternative therapies:

O Yoga

Yoga is an ancient Indian discipline that deals with the mind, body and spirit. This form of complementary therapy includes meditation and various physical postures. It also offers relaxation techniques. It is well-known to be a useful health accompaniment because it helps reduce pain, anxiety, and depression.

These three are symptoms of Fibromyalgia. Experts decided that Yoga could be an option for those suffering from the condition. Dr. James Carson, along with his associates, found that yoga can decrease the symptoms of Fibromyalgia and also improve one's personal function.

53 women took part in the study. The group included 25 women who participated in a "Yoga consciousness program."

Eight weeks of Yoga brought about significant improvement in participants' health. These women showed improvements in their moods, pain, fatigue and other symptoms of Fibromyalgia.

O Acupuncture

Acupuncture has been used for centuries in traditional Chinese medicine. It involves the placement of needles which target certain points. It is used in both eastern and western medicine. It has been proven to be effective in the treatment of nausea and vomiting.

Acupuncture also has been proven to alleviate Fibromyalgia symptoms according to current research. A 2006 study done by Dr. David Martin with associates revealed that people who had acupuncture reported lower levels of anxiety and fatigue, even seven months later.

Acupuncture is well-known for relieving pain. It is known that manipulating inserted needles can cause the release of endorphins, the body's natural painkillers.

Acupuncture can also alter brain chemistry. It alters the neurotransmitters release, which stops the chemical that transmit pain signals. This therapy can improve pain tolerance. The majority of chronic pain is relieved in a matter of weeks.

O Massage

Massage can be used to relieve stress, tension and pain. It involves the manipulation of muscles, tissues, and other body parts. It can increase blood circulation, and even enhance oxygenation if done correctly.

Massage can help reduce pain and stiffness. Additionally, it improves flexibility. Massage has been widely studied in Fibromyalgia. A 2009 study proved that massage could reduce pain and increase pain threshold. Additionally, massage can improve quality of living.

Here are some massage methods that have been found to benefit Fibromyalgia Patients:

Circulatory Massage – Uses deep pressure to ease tension and relieve pain.

Shiatsu – The manipulation of pressure points in the fingers and hands using the knuckles and fingers. It is very effective at relieving pain and relaxing the entire body.

o Reflexology – A technique that involves the manipulations of hands and toes. It has been found to ease pain, increase sleep, reduce fatigue, improve mental and physical health.

O Tai-chi

Tai-chi (or Tai Chi) is an ancient Chinese exercise that involves breathing control, meditation and gentle movements. It is based around the idea that a well-functioning mind will lead to a healthy and happy body. It has been used, over many years, to improve balance, flexibility, and muscular strength.

It is today considered to be one the best options for Fibromyalgia. It has been proven effective in relieving Fibromyalgia symptoms.

An expert study by Tufts University School of Medicine in 2010 backs this claim. The 12-week therapy involved the practice of 10 forms of Yang Style Tai-chi. The majority of the participants reported feeling less pain and more energy after the 12 week study.

O Chiropractic care

Chiropractic care can be described as a treatment option that relies on "the body, a self-healing organ." This means that the chiropractor adjusts your spine to alleviate widespread pain caused by Fibromyalgia.

It is one the most widely used complementary therapies for Fibromyalgia. Chiropractic care can help relieve pain. It has been shown to improve ranges and motion, particularly in the cervical spine.

The chiropractor will use gentle movement or pressure to maximize the body's curative properties. Sometimes, he may also perform high velocity stretches. He can increase the mobility of his spine, which might have been affected or restricted by Fibromyalgia.

Lifestyle Changes for Fibromyalgia Management

Fibromyalgia does not have a single cure. Lifestyle changes can help you manage your symptoms. These are some easy, yet profound lifestyle changes that can help to reduce Fibromyalgia symptoms.

O Eat healthy food

A poor diet can worsen Fibromyalgia symptoms. It is essential to eat a healthy diet.

You first have to improve your eating habits. These are some suggestions to help you remember.

o Choose high-fiber foods and low-fat foods.

o Consume lots of fruits, vegetables, grains. These fruits, vegetables and grains are rich in antioxidants that can fight cell-damaging free radicals. These elements are crucial because Fibromyalgia may be caused by oxidative damage.

Omega-3 Fatty Acids: Make it a habit to eat fatty fishes. They are also beneficial for the cardiovascular system and reduce swelling. These fatty acids are also known to help reduce stiffness, pain and stiffness.

Vitamin D supplementation can be helpful in relieving pain. Low levels can lead to an increase in the dosage of painkillers. Vitamin

D rich foods like beef liver, egg yolk, cheese and fatty fish are all good options for pain relief.

While there are foods that are healthy, there are foods that are not. Monosodium Glutamate(MSG), an additive found in Chinese food or sodas, can activate neuronal pathways that increase pain sensitivity. In fact, a study shows that cutting on MSG can reduce Fibromyalgia-associated pain.

O Exercise Regularly

Experts recommend that exercise be a key component in the treatment and prevention of Fibromyalgia. Regular physical activity can prevent muscle loss and decrease fatigue. It has also been shown to improve mental and physical well-being.

Patients should be encouraged to exercise regularly due to the many benefits it brings. Aerobics, flexibility programs and strength training are all important components of a good exercise routine.

Gradual Exercise is the most recommended program for Fibromyalgia. This program encourages physical activity to be gradually increased over time. The program starts with stretching exercises to relieve sore muscles and prevent future injury.

Following this, light exercise can be started. Swimming and walking are just two examples. The use of stationary bikes and treadmills is recommended. Once you have mastered the regimen, the intensity and duration of the exercises can be increased.

O Get sufficient sleep

Fibromyalgia symptoms include sleep disturbances. Sleep difficulties can cause more symptoms. Actually, those who cannot get restorative or good sleep often have worse symptoms.

Doctors recommend regular sleep habits to avoid sleep problems that can worsen Fibromyalgia. Follow these tips to achieve this.

o Don't drink too much fluids before going to bed, as this will help you avoid having a tendency to urinate in the early hours.

o Don't eat large meals prior to going to bed. A light snack is a good way to get sleep.

o Avoid alcohol and caffeine for 4 to 6 hours before going to sleep.

o Do not exercise more than 6 hours before bedtime. Your adrenaline could keep your awake at night.

o Do not take naps during the afternoon or night, as this can disrupt your sleep cycle.

O Reduce stress levels

Fibromyalgia sufferers tend to be more sensitive than others to stressful situations. Fibromyalgia can make it worse by increasing stress levels. It is possible to reduce stress and relieve symptoms.

There are many things that can be done to help with stress reduction. Good examples include:

* Biofeedback

Biofeedback, a treatment that reduces involuntary activities such as heart beat, blood pressure and skin temperatures, is called biofeedback. The idea behind biofeedback is to channel your mind and become more aware about your body. You will be able to take more control over your own health when you are more mindful of what is happening in your body. This method, as with other relaxation techniques can reduce pain.

Biofeedback is a form of electro-monitoring. The therapist will use flash and beep lights to monitor your heartbeat and muscle tension.

Once you have connected the equipment to your body, you can relax and do deep breathing. The therapist can also monitor your body as you do these things.

* Meditation

Meditation has been an effective relaxation technique for many millennia. Mindfulness Meditation is a well-known technique that Fibromyalgia patients use. Mindfulness meditation is a way to be conscious and open to all the thoughts that may come up in your head.

Fibromyalgia patients can benefit from meditation.

It can reduce pain. Meditation can lower Cortisol, which is a stress-causinghormone.

Better sleep Research shows that those who meditate are more likely to have higher levels Melatonin levels, which is a chemical that enhances sleep.

Higher well-being

Pace yourself

Fibromyalgia sufferers must be gentle with themselves. This is not about pushing yourself beyond the limits. This includes balancing activity and rest.

If you don't take care of your health, your symptoms will only get worse. Since symptoms are different from day to week, it is important that you keep your pace. Tomorrow you might not feel as good. It is important to be active.

Do not engage in any activities that are too exhausting. Although exercise can ease symptoms, excessive activity can cause them to worsen. The best way to improve your condition is to do the right activity at the right intensity. With time, your activities can be gradually increased in force.

Support For Fibromyalgia Patients

Do you feel as though you are the only one who understands your condition and you are completely alone? You don't have to worry because there are support groups that can help Fibromyalgia patient and their families. These associations are a good place to start if looking for a friend or a confidante.

NFA was founded 1997. This non-profit association is focused on supporting Fibromyalgia sufferers. For a nominal fee, interested parties can sign-up. NFA members get the latest updates on Fibromyalgia research.

Fibromyalgia Awareness Day is held annually by the NFA. Those with Fibromyalgia, as well as their family members, can take part in picnics, walks, and dinners. Fibromyalgia experts also share their expertise at conferences. It's not just a day of enjoyment, but it is also educational to help others learn more about this condition.

Fibromyalgia Network, which has been serving patients since 1998, offers research news and treatment. This website allows individuals to access Fibromyalgia articles that are informative as well the most current research.

You can also access many resources that will help you manage the disease. This website provides information and advice for Fibromyalgia patients, as well a list of consumer alerts.

This website has access to local support networks. Fibromyalgia Network provides a platform for you to connect with other people in similar situations, have empowering meetings and share your insights.

Chapter 4: The Placebo Effect

The beneficial effects of pain pills or injections that don't contain any active substance must also be addressed when we are discussing chronic pain. These inert compounds are known as placebo. Patients believe that they will be able to relieve pain by taking these pills or injections.

The placebo effect occurs quite often. The placebo effect is very common. It is believed that around one-third of people who use inactive substances will experience a relief in their pain. This effect can occur with different types pain such as toothache, arthritis pain, and even cancer pain. This placebo effect may be magnified by more intense therapeutic intervention. Surgery with its distinctive stigmas, scars and sutures can trigger a strong placebo effect. A well-known controlled research of arthroscopic surgical knee surgery, which is one of most common interventions to treat arthritic joint pain, has been published in New England Journal of Medicine 2002. Unbeknownstto them, a subset the 180 patients participated in a simulated operation. (These patients were put to sleep, but surgeons just made a small incision and stitched their knees. Patients who had real surgery felt as good as those who had it.

Because the placebo effect can be so prevalent, all scientific studies to determine if a drug has pain relief effectiveness must include a comparison group. The control group will, in theory, use the same pill/injection but will not contain any active ingredient. For a pain killer that is truly effective to be considered effective, it must make at least 30% more patients feel better. A positive relationship between the patient and their doctor can also have a placebo impact. It's been shown to improve patients' symptoms by simply explaining their diagnoses.

It is important to highlight certain characteristics of this placebo effect.

The effect does not have to be immediate. It can last for many months or even years.

The placebo effect can be experienced by everyone, not just those who are easily affected. The placebo effect is real because it releases the "internal pharmaceutical" of our body, namely many powerful internal painkillers called endorphins. We should forget that the placebo affect is "just our imagination" as patients who receive endorphin blocking drugs do not experience a placebo effect. But the placebo effect must not be taken to mean that there is no action. Contrary to popular belief. The placebo effect complements the effects and increases the effectiveness of medication.

Both physicians and patients should make use our powerful painkillers. This can only be done if there is a trusting and mutually understanding doctor-patient relationship.

Other than the placebo effect there are other natural causes chronic pain sufferers can experience an improvement in their condition after they take any substance. The first is that the condition is progressing in a normal way. The other reason is called regression to he mean. This means that symptoms will return to their normal state after an illness has reached a point in which they are exacerbated (e.g., when medication is given).

Summary

Placebo effect is the term for the beneficial pain-relief action that pills and injections without active ingredients can provide.

If you are convinced that a particular treatment will benefit your body, it releases its "internal pharmacy", which contains powerful painkillers called enorphins.

The placebo effect exists and can be achieved through good physician-patient relationships.

What is Stress?

Stress agents are any kind of stress agent that is either infectious, physical or emotional. This can all lead to the development of fibromyalgia. Understanding different concepts of stress is crucial. "Stress" is a confusing term. It is not a clear term. Other terms used to describe stress include "allostasis," "allostatic burden" and even "distress." Allostasis describes the additional effort needed to maintain balance when faced with more difficult situations. Allostatic burden is the price your body pays in order to adapt and thrive in an adverse environment.

It is important to remember that allostasis, stress, and distress have both physical and psychological connotations. Stressing agents include losing your job or divorce and even the death of a family member.

Fibromyalgia patients are frequently affected by stress, distress, or allostasis. People with fibromyalgia often deal with many of the above stressful situations. Depression and anxiety are two common symptoms. However, patients can experience stress themselves because they are rigid and perfectionist and obsessive about completing their work at work. They will sacrifice their lives to help those they love.

Summary

Stress can be defined as any stimuli - emotional or physical - that are designed to harm the balance and harmony of our body's functions.

Fibromyalgia may be caused by a constant attempt to adapt to stressful circumstances.

Our Stress Response System.

Amazing abilities animals have to adapt to constantly changing environmental conditions is a testament to their intelligence. If it is cold, the pores of our skin close instantly to maintain our body temperature constant. If the environment is very cold, the body will experience a shivering sensation that generates heat and maintains its temperature. In contrast, perspiration works to maintain internal body temperature when the surrounding environment is too warm. These responses to climate fluctuations are one example the incredible way the autonomic neurological system works. This system is responsible for internal regulation as well as adaptation to changes in the environment. This nervous is also responsible for responding in any way to stress. Because deregulation in the autonomic neuro system may be the key to fibromyalgia development, this chapter will outline the essential characteristics of this system.

The complex nervous network called the autonomic nervous systems is made up of many nerve cells that run through the body. They influence the functions and functioning of all the internal organs. The autonomic adjective means it acts independently from our will. It is also below the consciousness level. It is responsible to maintain basic vital functions (blood pressure and pulse rate), in harmony. These functions or parameters can be called vital signs. The function and functioning of every organ within the body, such as the heart or lungs, can be coordinated by this autonomic nervous system. It is responsible for responding to stressful situations. It activates the body's ability to respond to any threat. The autonomic nervous system works closely with the endocrine system (responsible for hormone production), especially with the hypothalamic-pituitary-adrenal axis. It also maintains a vital relationship with your immune system which, among other duties, is responsible for repelling diseases.

The brain stem and areas known as hypothalamus andthalamus contain the core of this autonomic nervous system. There are two branches of the autonomic nerve system. One could be called the accelerator. It is the sympathetic system that puts the body in a state of high alert, "ready for fight, flight" mode.

Adrenaline can be described as a hormone made in the adrenal glands. It is also called epinephrine. Because of its chemical formula, it belongs to a group known as catecholamines. This includes dopamine and norepinephrine. The true sympathetic transmitters are the two remaining. To avoid confusion, however, we will group them all under the familiar and generic term adrenaline.

The parasympathetic tree is the opposing branch to the sympathetic one. This branch has antagonistic actions that favor sleep, digestion, and other functions. This branch secretes most of the acetylcholine. Both branches are similar to yin and Yang: when sympathetic tone goes up, the natural result is a decline of parasympathetic voice.

The autonomic process follows a biological clock or the circadian rhythm. This means that each branch is active during day and night cycles. Daytime activity is predominately sympathetic. This allows the individual to be active and ready and able to react to everyday physical and intellectual demands. Parasympathetic activity can also be found at night, encouraging restful sleep. These night / day cycles are also followed closely by the hormone-producing endocrine system (mainly cortisol & melatonin).

A healthy animal and human body depends on maintaining a healthy circadian rhythm. Over thousands of centuries, night / day cycles followed the rhythms associated with external stimuli. This included light, noise and activity during daylight, darkness, silence and rest at night. Industrialization has dramatically altered these harmonious cycles. Light, noise, and activity all night can have an adverse effect on the functional balance in living beings.

The brain cortex is interconnected with our autonomic system. So emotions (rage or fear), which translate into biological responses such as paleness, dilation, tachycardia and tachycardia through sympathetic activation, are all part of the autonomic network. The interface between mind & body is the autonomic neurological system.

The autonomic neural system responds immediately. It's in charge of functions as simple and basic as keeping you from falling off the bed when you get up. When standing straight up, gravity tends to decrease blood circulation to the brain. Gravity alone could cause blood to accumulate in our legs' veins. The sympathetic system instantly makes adrenaline, which prevents blood pressure from dropping in the head. The heart beats more quickly and the blood vessels contract faster. Despite the force of gravity, this immediate reaction maintains brain water supply.

The sympathetic system is made up of branches that run along the spine and brain stem. These branches then travel to all organs in the chest or abdomen, particularly the heart and adrenal glands. The sympathetic system also functions in all four extremities. Parasympathetic is represented mainly in the vagus neuro that innervates heart and gastrointestinal systems.

The biological representation in Eastern philosophy of the concept of yin/yang is the autonomic neurological system. Yin Yang harmoniously unites opposites such as light and shadow and cold and heat. It also includes day and night, day and nights, moist and dry, and soft and hard. These are two opposites. But they are simultaneously dynamic, interdependent, and harmonious. Yin turns into Yang and vice versa. Yang is required to create Yin, and they together form Tao.

It was difficult to gauge the performance of such a highly variable system, as the activity of its two branches is constantly changing. "Heart Rate Variability Analysis" was created using advanced computer calculations in the eighties. This technology relies on the fact your heart rate changes in milliseconds. It is not fixed. Both branches of our autonomic nervous sistem, which are antagonistic but harmonious, control the periodic components. The parasympathetic section produces variations in heartbeat, which are coordinated with breathing. The sympathetic branch produces slower variations, which are due to monitors that constantly measure blood pressure. The computer can perform sophisticated analyses of the variability to determine the activity of each branch of the autonomic nervous systems. The benefit of this method is that all determinations are derived directly from EKG studies. Patients do not have to feel any discomfort.

A tilt stretcher, which is another way to study the function of the autonomous nervous system, is another option. A tilt stretcher that is horizontally tilted can be attached to people. This will allow them to see heart rate, blood pressure and blood pressure. Signs of

51

poor autonomic nervous function include excessive drops in bloodpressure, an increase in heart rates or fainting and a marked increase in blood pressure.

Summary

Living things have an inner yin/yang that balances our bodily functions. It is called the autonomous nervous system.

This system is also responsible to deal with stress.

It regulates the body's basic functions, such as blood pressure and breathing.

It is made up of two branches. An accelerator>> named sympathetic system works through the production adrenaline to alert the entire body.

Parasympathetic is the antagonist that favors sleep and digestion.

This system is in tune with the night/day cycles.

The autonomic neuro system is responsible for connecting mind and body functions.

The sympathetic branch manages stress response.

Two modern methods can be used to measure the performance of this system: heart rate variability analysis and tilt-table testing.

Fibromyalgia and its Manifestations

Genetic predisposition

Fibromyalgia can develop from a genetic predisposition. Different people can get the condition. We are one of several groups of researchers that has focused on the study genes that regulate the functions of the autonomic neural system. Specifically, we have studied the variations of the gene that yields the enzyme in charge of inactivating adrenaline, Cathecol-O-methyltransferase (COMT). As we will see, the study of this gene is important for two reasons. The first is that we believe that excessive adrenaline plays a major role in the onset of fibromyalgia. Zwei separate research groups discovered that certain gene variations produce an enzyme called "lazy", which is unable to properly breakdown adrenaline. It also makes people feel intense pain stimuli. This means that people who lack adequate adrenaline clearance from their bodies are more vulnerable to being persistently in pain.

Turkish researchers have discovered that patients with Fibromyalgia suffer from a less frequent variation in the COMT genes. Garcia-Fructuoso, the Catalonian physician, joined our efforts to determine if there were any genetic variations in the COMT genes in patients with Fibromyalgia. However, we did not find a strong correlation between Mexican and Spanish women. Another study looked at genetic variations of adrenaline receptors. In this study, we found that both Spanish and Mexican patients with fibromyalgia had a genetic makeup linked to defects in adrenaline.

We should stress that genetic alterations are not the cause of fibromyalgia. Genetic alteration does not cause this disease.

Previous episodes

It is common for people suffering from fibromyalgia, to say that they have felt vague discomfort for years before experiencing the onset or diffuse pain. Some recall feeling tired since childhood and complaining of pain in their legs and arms as children. They say that their teenager classmates were able to stay up late and get up early the next morning in order to practice sports. But, future patients feel "beaten" and are unable or unwilling to keep up with their friends.

Factors to trigger Fibromyalgia

It is possible for the condition to manifest after a defined stressful event. For example, a serious injury to the spine or severe physical trauma. Fibromyalgia patients often have a "whiplash," as a result from a car crash. A third of patients with fibromyalgia experience physical trauma.

Fibromyalgia has been linked to several infections. Lyme disease is caused by an unusual bacteria called the spirochete. Fibromyalgia can also be caused by viruses that are not yet well understood. Other potential triggers include: emotional trauma, including the death or serious injury of a family member, physical and mental abuse, as well as constant, intense, extreme, or prolonged, repetitive, physical effort such that competitive sports are required, or harassment at work.

Other environmental factors

The ongoing study of a large population of British Isles-born people in 1958 has helped to identify factors that could lead to chronic, generalized pain. According to the British study, unhealthy lifestyles are also associated with persistent pain. Chronic pain is linked to unhealthy lifestyle choices, such as obesity, smoking and eating fats. While this English study does not identify how many people suffer from chronic pain, it is important to note that other epidemiological studies in people with fibromyalgia also support the association. An unhealthy diet, obesity or smoking are all associated with the development and/or worsening of the disease. Syndromes similar to Fibromyalgia can develop in combatants of different armed conflicts. This was clearly demonstrated during the Persian Gulf War. After serving in conflict, many British and US volunteers developed the so called "gulfwar syndrome".

Summary

Recent studies reveal that pain intensity perceptions can be genetically coded.

Individuals with the COMT enzyme are immune to pain. This enzyme breaks down adrenaline efficiently.

The ability of the COMT gene to produce the enzyme is determined by its punctual variation.

It is less common for patients suffering from Fibromyalgia to be able to identify the COMT-producing genes that efficiently reduce adrenaline.

In a subgroup, fibromyalgia can be caused by severe trauma.

This disease can also be triggered if there is emotional trauma or an infection.

Chronic pain can result from eating junk food and smoking, as well as being overweight.

The primary complaint is generalized pain

All patients with Fibromyalgia experience different levels of pain. Patients who visit their doctors complain of intense pain. On a scale of 1-10 (where 10 represents the most intense pain an individual can experience) 7 is the average level of pain that fibromyalgia patients feel when they visit their doctor for help. It can be experienced all over the body. However, most people feel it in the joints, muscles and bones. This symptom may be more severe in the neck and lower back than it is in the legs.

There are many factors that affect pain. These include changes in weather, menstrual cycles, sleep quality and emotional tension. It is possible to experience little discomfort for several days or weeks. However, it is the hardest time of day for most patients. Many patients wake up feeling like they've been "beaten."

The most significant characteristic of fibromyalgia-related pain is its presence with abnormal sensations within the limbs. These sensations are called paresthesias by doctors. They include tingling or burning sensations and discomfort in tight clothes. Paresthesias provide important information that helps distinguish between fibromyalgia from pain caused by other rheumatic ailments.

Patients also have headaches as a result of their generalized suffering. The pain may be diffused or could have the characteristics of migraine. It usually affects one side and is accompanied sometimes by nausea and sensitivity.

Summary

Fibromyalgia's most prevalent manifestation is generalized or chronic pain. It may cause a variety of unpleasant sensations including pricking/burning, stinging and cramps.

Other Frequent Manifestations

Apart from chronic pain, fibromyalgia patients can experience many symptoms. Although not all complaints will be present in every case of fibromyalgia, they are more common than in other forms of rheumatic disease. Patients shouldn't be concerned about the detailed explanations that follow. They are only meant to inform patients of all possible signs.

Fatigue

The most common sign of Fibromyalgia and a constant symptom is tiredness. Resting does not help. Patients wake up feeling tired or worse than before going to sleep. Plus, they are often exhausted from their daily activity. Patients feel that they are running out of fuel or that their batteries have run dry by the time they get to work in the morning. There is a commonality between fibromyalgia, chronic fatigue syndrome, and others as we will see.

Unrestful sleep

Sleep disturbances include frequent awakenings, or wakefulness during the night. EEG studies show that patients with Fibromyalgia have a longer time to reach stage 4, and for shorter periods. Stage 4 sleep has delta waves dominating and generating deep, refreshing, restful sleep. The intrusions by alpha waves can interrupt deep sleep, causing fibromyalgia patients to wake up. Researchers have conducted experiments on healthy subjects to see if deep sleep could be interrupted by shaking them or making them listen to loud noises. After several days, the patients experienced symptoms similar to fibromyalgia.

Mental fog

Some people feel bewildered and have difficulty concentrating or thinking clearly. This is called "fibro fog". The patient may have memory problems, which can make it difficult to remember what product to buy at the grocery store. Sometimes patients have trouble finding the right words. These symptoms do not indicate an early sign of Alzheimer's disease.

Dryness in the mouth or eyes

Eyes can feel dry and itchy, while the mouth can feel dry. These symptoms are also typical in Sjogren's syndrome. Sjogren's is different because the dryness is caused by inflammation of glands that produce saliva and tears.

Painful palpitations near the heart

These symptoms may raise concerns for patients as they indicate the presence of a serious heart condition. The patient may feel pain and pricking at the heart. They might also feel a strong pulse.

Dizziness, fainting

The most common symptom is dizziness, which rarely causes fainting. These alterations could be caused by low blood pressure that is common in certain cases. A buzzing sound in the ears or hypersensitivity may also occur.

Irritable bowel syndrome

This condition affects approximately 30% to 50%. It's characterized as abdominal distension with colic or increased intestinal gas. There is constipation at times, and sometimes diarrhea. A stool analysis does not reveal any signs or symptoms of infection.

Hands are cold and bluish

Raynaud phenomena is a phenomenon that results in a constriction of blood vessels in the hands, and feet, when the temperature drops. They become "corpse hands", and within minutes turn from waxy white to purple, then finally to red. Raynaud's phenomenon can be seen in patients with fibromyalgia. This is what happens when small blood vessels dilate constantly. This is why your hands feel damp, cold and bluish.

Temporomandibular joints syndrome

This condition, in which patients experience pain and spasms around the mandibular bone and teeth grinding at night, is something dentists are familiar with. Bruxism is the term used to describe this condition. It can be hard to open your mouth and eat.

Non-infectious Cystitis

Patients frequently have to get up several times per night to urinate. They void small amounts of urine. It is very common for patients to feel a strong urge to go to their bathroom. Violating is painful and can sting. While this may indicate an infection or a bacterial problem, these urine cultures prove to be persistently negative. Interstitial cystitis is the other type of cystitis.

Vaginal pain

Itching, burning, and/or constant pain are common in this area. It is possible that there may be an infectious cause. If you experience discomfort that is similar to menstruation, it may be endometriosis. Sometimes, sexual intercourse can cause pain.

Endometriosis

Endometriosis can be caused by the endometrium (the tissue that lines your womb) becoming lodged in other parts such as the bladder, the eggs, or the rectum. Endometriosis, which can occur during menstruation, can cause cramps and pelvic pain. It can also lead to pain during sexual intercourse, after a bowel movements, and other symptoms. Endometriosis is a common cause of infertility and affects young women. Fibromyalgia is more common for women with endometriosis.

Restless leg syndrome

This is a painful feeling in the legs that causes pain and makes it difficult to move. Some symptoms include involuntary or uncontrollable jerking of the lower legs. In some cases, iron deficiencies have been identified. Another characteristic is the favorable response to LDopa-containing medication for Parkinson's disease. Recent discoveries have revealed a mutation in Chromome 6p21.2 that may be related to this syndrome. This shows there is clearly a genetic predisposition.

Immune alterations

Fibromyalgia sufferers can experience different allergic reactions. Candida can also cause yeast infections (mainly vaginal) in some cases.

Psychological impact

Fibromyalgia can cause anxiety. Patients feel anxious, uneasy, and unable or unwilling to relax. There is often depression, sadness, and dismay. It is hard to know if anxiety or depression are the causes or effects of Fibromyalgia. It's better to be pragmatic and accept the truth. These patients may suffer from anxiety/depression. The disease and the condition deserve medical attention. In severe cases of depression, professional treatment may be necessary. Panic attack, another psychological problem linked to fibromyalgia, is also a possibility. Patients can experience panic attack episodes, feeling uncontrollable fear and the sense that they are at risk of suffering a serious psychological problem.

Signs during the physical examination

There is often a sharp contrast between the symptoms and abnormalities patients report and the intensity and variety they experience. Many physicians are confused by the disease and might be tempted to tell patients, after they have done a physical exam, that there's nothing wrong. However, it is possible for discrete alterations to be recognized. The most fundamental of these, according to classical criteria, is tenderness when palpating in certain well defined anatomical points.

The exact location of 18 points is shown in the following image: Fibromyalgia. There are 9 points per side, making a total 18.

1. Occipital- In the back section of the skull, from where the muscles of the occipital region originate.

2. Lower cervical spine at the site for the transverse process of vertebrae 5-7 (C5-7.

3. Trapezius, located in the middle of trapezius' muscle.

4. Supraspinatus muscle- at the upper, inner border of scapula. Here is where supraspinatus muscle arises.

5. Second rib: At the junction of the second bone and the sternum.

6. Lateral epicondyle- on the bony prominences in the humerus.

7. Gluteus-on the upper external quadrants of the gluteus.

8. Greater Trochanter: The bony prominence of a femur is what makes it the Greater Trochanter

9. Kneel on the Medial Fat Pad

These sites are not actually points of information. This is because you can apply pressure to any part or body of the body with a force which normally would not trigger any pain. Allodynia refers to this increased sense of touch.

Other, less common but related to fibromyalgia, alterations can be discovered during the physical exam. Low blood pressure is possible in patients with fibromyalgia. The systolic level should be below 100 millimeters.

Although the alteration is not visible, it is essential in diagnosingfibromyalgia. Because of the contrast between white skin and the fine bluish web created by the superficial veins, people with fair skin can easily see it. This phenomenon, known liveo reticularis is more prominent in cold weather.

There is a link between excessive joint movement and fibromyalgia. This can be more noticeable in adolescents. In such cases, girls may touch the palmar portion of their forearms using their thumbs, or bend backwards. They can also bend forward so that their entire palm rests on the floor, but not bend their knees.

Negative results from physical examinations are crucial to confirm the diagnosis.

Summary

A majority of patients with Fibromyalgia complain that they feel tired and irritable.

Physical examination shows that there is an over-sensitive skin to pressure in multiple places. 18 anatomical points are considered sensitive to pressure.

What Do Laboratory Tests Say?

All lab tests result are normal, so it is easy to summarize. Physicians who don't know much about fibromyalgia will use this argument to assure the patient that nothing is wrong.

It is important to check that the patient with fatigue has not been anemic. Also, certain immune alterations like antinuclear and rheumatoid genes (or rheumatoid) should be checked. If there are any immune alterations, this would indicate the presence of an autoimmune disorder such as Sjogren's Syndrome, Rheumatoid Arthritis, or Lupus

Erythematosus. We will talk later about how these pathologies can be misdiagnosed as fibromyalgia.

It is also important to ensure that test results for thyroid gland function fall within the normal limits. Thyroid dysfunction (either poor or excessive) is a reason for fatigue. Additionally, there is a correlation between chronic pain and the presence of antithyroid antibodies. It is important to confirm that laboratory tests showing inflammation (especially erythrocyte sedimentation rate or C-reactive Protein) are not altered.

Although MRI or Xray images may not show any obvious abnormalities, it is possible to confuse the situation. Normal images can show signs of wear or bulging between the vertebrae in normal subjects after the age 40. Sophism is not uncommon.

The patient complains that he or she is experiencing neck pain.

(r. X ray or MRI) images of this area show wear.

The wear of the cervical spinal column can cause pain.

In cases of lower back discomfort, the same error can occur. If fibromyalgia sufferers also feel a burning, tingling sensation in their limbs, this could falsely indicate that wear is causing nerve root compression. Therefore, such patients may require surgery to either the cervical spine or the back. Chronic pain in different areas of the body is an indication that people suffering from fibromyalgia need to be treated more often and less frequently. This is why both doctors and patients must be aware of the disease. There is a flip side to this, however. Fibromyalgia does NOT make a person immune to other conditions. If there is a change in the pattern of symptoms, physicians should also be alert for this possibility.

Summary

There is no lab test that can confirm the presence of Fibromyalgia.

It is important that you confirm that there are not any other causes for your pain and/or fatigue.

Atypical X-ray findings should be treated with caution since bone wear occurs after the age of 40.

Patients suffering from fibromyalgia need to be rehabilitated more frequently because of chronic pain.

Chapter 5: How Fibromyalgia Is Diagnosed

Because fibromyalgia may be confused with other diseases, it can make it difficult to identify. There is also the "fibromyalgia-profile", which is defined as having chronic, severe pain for more than 3 months. It can be confused with other diseases. It is important to confirm the presence of pain with pressure on any anatomical components mentioned earlier, and that all laboratory tests have returned normal results. If all the criteria are met, it will likely be fibromyalgia.

The American College of Rheumatology approved new criteria in 2010 for diagnosing fibromyalgia. These guidelines, apart from being cumbersome, remain controversial because they neglect an essential part of the diagnostic process, namely the physical exam. These criteria are unable to recognize fibromyalgia, a real illness, as they do not consider it a valid diagnosis. Finally, it is important to mention that Dr Wolfe, a respected researcher and leader of the group that developed these criteria, has said that fibromyalgia cannot be considered a valid diagnosis. It seems paradoxical that diagnostic guidelines should be proposed for a condition already ruled out. These new guidelines are only going to be of real value when time allows.

Below is information about the 2010 controversial standards:

If these 3 conditions are met then a patient has met the diagnostic criteria of fibromyalgia.

1. Widespread discomfort index (WPI), equal/more 7 and symptom severity scale (SS), scale score equal/more 5 or WPI 3 to 6 and SSscale score equal/more 9.

2. You have had symptoms at a similar level for at most 3 months.

3. The pain is not due to a condition.

Assessment: WPI: Note the number of places where the patient had pain during the week. How many areas have the patients experienced pain? Score will be between 0 - 19. Score will be between 0 to 19.

SS score: Fatigue, waking tired, cognitive symptoms

Each of the three symptoms listed above should be indicated using the following scale.

0 = no problem

1 = Very minor or minor problems. Generally, mild to intermittent.

2 = moderate or substantial problems that are often present, and/or at a moderate degree

3 = severe: pervasive, continuous, life-disturbing problems

You can determine whether the patient has somatic symptoms by looking at them in general.

0 = not feeling any symptoms, 1 = not feeling any symptoms, 2 = mild symptoms, 3 = quite a few symptoms

The SS Score is the sum of the 3 symptoms (fatigue; waking unrefreshed; cognitive symptoms) along with the severity (or extent or severity) of all other symptoms. The final score will range between 0 and 12.

These are some of the possible symptoms: muscle pain, irritable intestinal syndrome, fatigue/tiredness. Itching, brain or memory problems.

Summary

Fibromyalgia can sometimes be hard to diagnose. Many other diseases can also be confused with fibromyalgia.

To determine it is present, you will need to look for signs such as generalized chronic pain, hypersensitivity to pressure in different areas of the body and other symptoms.

The 2010 release of new diagnostic criteria to diagnose fibromyalgia was controversial.

Fibromyalgia is Not the Only Disease You Can Confront

Because they can also cause pain or fatigue, there are a few diseases that may be confused with fibromyalgia.

Rheumatoid Arthritis

It's another common rheumatic disease, which affects about 1%. Most of these cases are women. It causes swelling in multiple areas and morning stiffness. Laboratory tests have shown that 90% of cases are affected by rheumatoid and/or anti-cyclic citrullinated antibodies. Rheumatoid arthritis can be disabling if not treated properly. The disease can gradually erode your joints. It is necessary to determine whether there is ostensible swelling at multiple joints in order to make a differential diagnosis. People suffering from fibromyalgia may feel that their joints and hands are swollen, as we've already noted.

Lupus Erythematosus

This condition is also more prevalent in younger women. It is also included in the list of auto-immune conditions. (This indicates that the immune system is hyperactive and attacks elements of the body as foreign. This disease may also have multiple manifestations. There is joint pain, but it has less swelling than rheumatoid. Rash can develop on the cheeks. This is known as the "butterflywing" pattern. Sensitivity to sunlight can cause skin irritations and fever in some patients. Some cases may result in kidney damage due to proteinuria. The condition may also cause inflammation in membranes that surround the lungs or heart. Lupus can also lead to fatigue.

Laboratory tests may reveal anemia and a decline among a certain subset of leucocytes known as lymphocytes. Sometimes false positives can be detected by the VDRL testing for syphilis. Antinuclear antibodies can be found in nearly every case. This makes the test extremely important in identifying patients with lupus. An important clarification is required here. Although the antinuclear allergy test is highly sensitive, it can also detect antinuclear immune reactions in people with other conditions, including fibromyalgia. Lupus is a condition where antinuclear immunity is visible even when serum has been diluted several times. Besides, lupus is home to specific antibodies, such as anti-DNA, anti–Sm, anti–Ro/SSA/SSB and anti–RNP. In contrast, antinuclear substances in fibromyalgia can only be found at low dilutions, and they are not specific.

The problem of confusing Lupus with Fibromyalgia is real. It's not unusual for patients to be treated for Lupus, but they are actually suffering from fibromyalgia. The confusion comes because both conditions affect women and can cause diffuse pain, fatigue and other heterogeneous effects such as joint pains. The two diseases could have antinuclear immunoglobulins. But the fundamental difference is that lupus damages the body's structure. Lupus also affects internal organs like kidneys and hematologic system, resulting in low lymphocyte counts or anemia. Fibromyalgia however does not harm the body structure. As previously mentioned, there are antinuclear antibodies in Lupus. However, fibromyalgia does not have any specificity.

This confusion between Lupus fibromyalgia and Lupus can get even more complicated when we consider that both diseases are interrelated. That is, patients can have both diseases simultaneously. It is vital to establish if such an association exists. Fibromyalgia symptoms may not indicate that lupus cannot be controlled. Cortisone can make symptoms worse.

Polymyalgia Rheumatica

Even the name of the condition resembles fibromyalgia. Polymyalgia has a common occurrence in people over 50. It causes diffuse pain, mostly in the neck or lumbar region, and significant morning muscle stiffness. Lab tests for inflammation in this instance are different from fibromyalgia. In this case, the C-reactive factor is altered. Erythocyte sedimentation rates are often greater than 50 mm/hr. Another difference is the fact that symptoms of polymyalgia are usually onset in weeks or even months. Fibromyalgia however, can start many years earlier.

Another distinction is the striking response of polymyalgia-rheumatica when given low doses of cortisone. This contrasts with the lackluster response in fibromyalgia. In certain cases, the therapeutic test can be used to identify between the two conditions.

Spondyloarthritis

Spondyloarthritis affects mostly young males. The spine becomes more fused as the disease progresses. Ankylosing spondylitis is the diagnosis. These conditions cause lower back and joint pains, as well as inflammation and tendonitis in the legs. Patients report feeling stiff and numb the next day. Women tend to feel more affected by spondyloarthitis. Pain in the neck can be more prominent in women. Examining spinal radiographs can be used to determine if you have spondyloarthitis. The sacroiliac joint is located in the posterior part. HLA B27, a laboratory test to help differentiate between the two types of conditions, is available. Most people with spondyloarthitis receive positive results. One difference is that the pain associated with spondyloarthitis typically improves when anti-inflammatory medication is used. This is unlike fibromyalgia.

Gluten Intolerance

Gluten is a form of glycoprotein found within the seeds of many cereals. It is made up two components: glutenin, and gliadin. Gliadin could be immunotoxic, which can lead to a host of other diseases in the susceptible. Celiac disease, which usually develops in infancy, causes persistent diarrheal and delayed growth. Celiac illness often disappears when you eat gluten-free. A diagnosis of Celiac disease can be confirmed by testing antibodies against gliadin/endomysium//or transglutaminase. Endoscopy reveals atrophy of intestinal villi and chronic inflammation in testine biopsies.

Adults who are gluten intolerant can develop other symptoms that may be mistakenly referred to as fibromyalgia. Although diarrhea is not always apparent, patients can also experience headaches, dizziness or depression. It is important that you distinguish this condition from fibromyalgia. As stated previously, gluten intolerance often improves with the elimination of it from the diet.

Nerve Trunk Compression

The nerves that control different sensations to brain come from the spine. They travel through inter-vertebral cavities and along the limbs until they reach the hands or feet. They can cause pain and discomfort in the areas they are active if they become compressed close together. The carpal tunnel is a narrow channel that runs through the wrists and can cause nerve compression. Tingling is experienced in the first three hands. Fibromyalgia is also known for causing pain and burning. This is why it is common for patients to misunderstand whether they are undergoing surgery to remove the carpal tunnel or to correct the cervical spine. These operations can result in poor results. Avoid these mistakes by keeping the following things in mind. It is important to identify if there are any symptoms that could be caused by a compressed nerve root. Inspect the electrodemyography and nerve conduction velocity for signs of compression. Find out if the individual is suffering from fibromyalgia.

Arnold-Chiari Malformation

This malformation occurs when the cerebellum is compressed in the orifice, which connects with the skull. This causes weakness in the arms and tingling. It is possible for gait to be irregular and there may be pain in the neck, head and neck. The physical exam can sometimes reveal a change in the inferior brain nerves. This may be interpreted as an abrogation of the gag reflex. It is common to see weakness and atrophy within the muscles of your arm, along with diminished reflexes. Babinski sign refers specifically to abnormal reflexes in the feet.

The diagnosis is confirmed by magnetic resonance imaging, (MRI) at base of the cranium that shows settling in the cervical amygdalae and compression leading to the cervical spine.

One group of patients was diagnosed with Fibromyalgia. However, after thorough examination it was determined that they had Arnold-Chiari malformation. They experienced relief from their symptoms by having their craniums removed. These anecdotal cases caused a lot concern among some neurosurgeons from the United States. Some stories published by mass communication media stated that surgery on a portion of the cranium could treat fibromyalgia. However, many patients were forced to take unnecessary risks.

It is essential to distinguish fibromyalgia form Arnold-Chiari misformation using careful clinical examination and, if appropriate, MRI.

In all of the conditions above, pain is the primary symptom and source of confusion for fibromyalgia. A combination of fibromyalgia or other diseases can lead to intense fatigue. This is a listing of the most important.

Sjogren's Syndrome

This is a common rheumatic disorder and is similar to Lupus. Sjogren's syndrome's most prominent characteristic is dryness in the mouth, eyes, and throat. These symptoms are very common in fibromyalgia. As we have seen, they are also frequent in Sjogren's syndrome. However, the chronic inflammation of salivary glands and tears causes dryness in Sjogren's. Biopsies from the inner lip glands can confirm the inflammation. Sjogren's Syndrome can also cause fatigue or joint pain. Lab tests are often positive for rheumatoid and antinuclear antibodies. These include anti–La/SSB, anti-Ro/SSA, or anti–La/SSA. Sjogren's Syndrome and fibromyalgia can co-occur, just like lupus. Patients with fibromyalgia who use antidepressants are likely to have dry mucosal surfaces.

Multiple sclerosis is in its early stages

Multiple sclerosis can be described as a disease that causes inflammation to the brain and spine cord. It leaves scarring throughout the nervous system. Myelin, a protein that protects and cushions the nerves, is affected. Multiple sclerosis can cause fatigue, but also abnormal sensations, and localized weakness in the legs. In the initial stages, MS can lead to confusion with fibromyalgia. This happens when there is intense fatigue.

Thyroid gland function changes

In this situation, fatigue can manifest in one of two ways: when there is too many thyroid hormones (hyperthyroidism), and when there are fewer (hypothyroidism). Thyroid function tests should be used to check for proper gland function in all patients with fibrimyalgia.

Hypoglycemia in the adrenal glands

This is a rare condition that causes an insufficient amount of cortisone to be produced by the adrenal glands. First, it is important to know that the adrenal cells (located above the kidneys) contain two components. They are the cortex that produces cortisone or the medulla of adrenaline. People with impaired adrenal cortex function may experience fatigue, weight loss, and chronic weakness. Sometimes they have pigmentation issues and their blood pressure can be low. There are many things that may be connected with fibromyalgia. An adrenal gland defect can be distinguished with fibromyalgia. The discomforts have a shorter development and there is no internal cortisone.

Chronic infection by the hepatitis-type C virus

Indolent liver inflammation is the result of this virus. It is most often transmitted by infected bloodtransfusions, but it can also transmit through contaminated injectable drug addicts' syringes. It is sometimes transmitted by tattoo-related instruments that aren't sterilized. The virus is less likely to be transmitted through blood transfusions than before, as there are specific tests for detecting it.

Extreme fatigue can result from chronic hepatitis C infection. Most cases have altered liver function tests. It is crucial to look into any history of blood transfusions and tattoos.

Vitamin D deficiency

Vitamin D deficiencies are very common in the population. Common causes include inadequate intake, insufficient absorption, intestinal diseases, and not enough sunlight exposure. Normal levels of vitamin A in blood range from 30 to 75 nanograms per million. Patients suffering from fibromyalgia are more likely to have vitamin D deficiencies than those with less outdoor activity. However, only a small number of cases of fibromyalgia (below 10 nanograms/milliliter) may respond to chronic vitamin-D supplementation. It is a good idea to check the blood levels if someone with fibromyalgia lives a life that may indicate a vitamin deficiency.

Medication-related pain in the joints or muscles

Many drugs can cause pain in the muscles. Due to their frequentity, statins (which are used for high levels of cholesterol) and aromatase inhibitions used in breast cancer treatment are both important.

Statins may cause muscle weakness or pain. Laboratory tests frequently reveal elevated levels of creatine Kinase (muscle enzyme) in the blood.

Joint pain is common in up to 60% people who take aromatase inhibitors for breast-cancer. This can make it difficult to function.

Muscle and/or joint pains caused by medication disappear after a few weeks or months.

In this chapter we've seen how difficult it can become to distinguish fibromyalgia form other diseases that can cause similar discomforts. We want to stress that the problem doesn't end there. The flip side of the coin must be seen. Fibromyalgia is a condition that can manifest in many ways. It does not give immunity to the possibility of developing other conditions. Fibromyalgia patients need to be examined by a physician familiar with all aspects of internal medicine.

Summary

There are many conditions that could be confused with Fibromyalgia.

Contrary fibromyalgia is not the only disease that can cause inflammation or visible damage to your body's structures.

There are many drugs available that can cause muscular pain.

People may experience fibromyalgia or another rheumatic diseases simultaneously.

Before you are able to undergo surgery to reduce the pressure on the nerve root and the carpal canal, fibromyalgia should be excluded.

Conditions That Are Inextricably Related to Fibromyalgia

There are many syndromes, which is the term used to describe a series of symptoms that present in the same way as fibromyalgia. We have already talked about several diseases that can be found in certain parts of the body such as irritable stool syndrome, temporomandibular, and noninfectious cystitis. Now we will talk about others that share many of the same characteristics as fibromyalgia. These diseases may also have similar development mechanisms. We will be talking about myalgic fatigue syndrome, chronic fatigue syndromes, myalgic neuropathy, the Gulf War syndromes, multiple chemical sensitivity and reflex sympathetic dystrophy as well as post-polio symptoms.

Myalgic and chronic fatigue syndrome are now known as myalgic or myalgic.

This is the result of severe chronic fatigue, lasting for at least six months. It cannot be explained by other diseases. Fatigue does not improve when you rest and can cause significant impairments in the ability to function. According to current diagnostic criteria patients who suffer from fatigue must show at least four out of eight of the following symptoms.

1. Muscle pain

2. Joint pain

3. Sore throat

4. Swollen neck ganglia, sensitive to palpation

5. Memory and concentration

6. Headaches

7. You feel uneasy after working out

8. Unrestful sleep

It is clear that the symptoms are very similar to fibromyalgia. Since four of eight minor criteria are related to pain, one can easily see the similarities. There are subtle differences between chronic fatigue syndrome and fibromyalgia, making them more likely to have an underlying viral infection. Chronic fatigue syndrome can cause feverish symptoms, as well as persistent activation or activation of our defense system. This is why many of the investigations that have been undertaken to investigate this entity focused on finding a specific virus. Experts say that fibromyalgia (and chronic fatigue syndrome) are very different conditions. Most people with fibromyalgia fall under the definition of chronic fatigue syndrome if they are applied to current classification criteria. The most important difference between these two syndromes is in the level and intensity of the main discomfort.

There seems a common understanding among various groups of patients with chronic fatigue syndrome, as well scholars. It is thought that the use of the name chronic tired syndrome trivializes this condition and makes it seem normal. A group of experts on the subject met in 2007 and proposed myalgic or myalgic to be the name for this entity. It is highly probable that the term chronic fatigue disorder will soon be forgotten.

Gulf War Syndrome

The Gulf War Syndrome is an intriguing pathology in the investigation of fibromyalgia. Both the United States, and the United Kingdom, sent youths (mostly boys) to Iraq during the 1991 war in the Persian Gulf. These young recruits were healthy and strong, and their health was confirmed by strict military medical exams. After returning from war, one third developed a chronic disease that was often debilitating and disabling. The most prominent symptoms were severe fatigue, muscle, joint pain, difficulty in concentration, memory problems, fever, and diarrhea. Initial reports dismissed the condition as "nervousness from stress." However, more recent research has shown that there were changes in the neuronal system similar to those seen in fibromyalgia. While it is possible that troops were exposed, the theory of an autonomic nerve system alteration that triggered the disease remains unconfirmed. This is critical for fibromyalgia research. These details allow us to better understand the causes and symptoms.

Multiple Chemical Sensitivity

This is called hypersensitivity to chemical or environment agents. It causes skin, respiratory, digestive and psychological irritation. It is believed that different artificial chemicals irritate more sensitive areas of your body. Fernandez Sola et. al. have determined that the most common sensitizers are organic fuel byproducts, solvents (solvents), as well as phosphorated chemicals (insecticides). Itchy skin, irritation to the nose and throat, fatigue, weakness, muscle pain, nausea, vomiting, diarrhea, dullness, fatigue, headaches, and itchy eyes may be caused by low levels of some of these agents. Eliminating sensitizer substances may improve symptoms.

Reflex Sympathetic Dystrophy has been renamed complex regional pain disorder

The syndrome develops usually after trauma to an arm or leg. After a few weeks, patients may feel a burning sensation on one limb, with intense palpation and swelling. These discomforts are persistent. The affected limb may begin to lose strength over time. The burning sensation may sometimes be felt on another limb.

It has been proven that the sympathetic traffic of the damaged limb is increased and that blocking the sympathetic pathways reduces this pain. Reflex sympathetic disorder is an example that the sympathetic system maintains pain. It has many similarities to fibromyalgia as well, as we'll see. We believe that fibromyalgia might be a form of generalized reflex sympathetic dystrophy. This condition is known today as "complex local pain syndrome".

Post-Polio Syndrome

Post-polio is another condition similar to Fibromyalgia. Polio was a terrible condition that affected many children around the world in the second half the 20th century. It is caused due to a virus. The virus damages the nerve cell of the spinal chord that controls the commands to the muscles. Children with polio were paralysed and suffered progressive atrophy in their legs and arms. In some cases, respiratory muscles became paralyzed and could even lead to death. There are many serious side effects of polio, including weakness in the legs and flaccidness.

The vaccine against polio, which was developed by doctors Salk (and Sabin) in the latter half of the 20th Century, is undoubtedly one the most amazing and undisputed successes of modern scientific medicines. This vaccine effectively eradicated the deadly illness.

It has been seen that patients with polio have atrophy and weakness in the muscles for many decades. This can be accompanied by severe fatigue, diffuse pain in joints and muscles similar to those experienced in fibromyalgia.

The exact cause of post-polio is still unknown. There is speculation that the post-polio syndrome may cause muscular weakness and atrophy relapses because the spinal nerves which resisted the original attack to polio grew to compensate for the lost function. This growth happens at the neuromuscular plaque, the place where the nerve joins the muscular. The nerves that are enlarged eventually give up, causing weakness in the muscles.

Summary

There are a variety of diseases similar to fibromyalgia.

Fibromyalgia can share many characteristics with myalgic encephalopathy or chronic fatigue syndrome.

The Trueness and Beauty of Pain

It is crucial to establish if the pain the patient feels is real or imagined before you can discuss the development of fibromyalgia.

Some researchers believe that fibromyalgia pain is imaginary, despite the fact that there isn't any evidence of damage to the pain sites (muscles/joints/ligaments) and normal lab tests. Recent and more extensive investigations confirm that this pain is real.

Many research groups have shown that the cerebrospinal water of patients with fibromyalgia has high levels of an element called substance "P". The cerebrospinal water is contained in the central neurological system. It directly bathes every structure of the brain. Substance P acts as the pain transmitter. It accumulates in dorsal root Ganglia (the spinal cord). Its primary function, however, is to amplify painful sensations.

Also, it has been shown that patients with fibromyalgia have very high levels in their cerebrospinal water. This element is called nerve growth fact. In animal models, this growth hormone induces persistent painful behavior. However, more importantly it causes structural changes to the dorsal Root

Ganglia with budding and activation of the sympathetic terminals. As mentioned in Chapter 3, dorsal nerve ganglia act as the main centers of pain modulation.

Initial clinical trials showed that the nerve growth factors could be used as a treatment to Alzheimer disease. However, tests were stopped after patients experienced severe back pain.

Another evidence supporting the veracity pain is provided by brain imaging methods. Functional magnetic resonance image (fMRI), was used in order to prove that even stimuli that are not usually painful, can trigger brain centers that sense pain.

There is now strong evidence to support the claim that fibromyalgia-related pain is real. Once that fact has been established, it's time to find the cause of the pain.

Summary

There is overwhelming evidence that fibromyalgia pain exists.

The cerebrospinal fluid comes in close contact with your brain. It contains high levels, in fact, of substances that cause pain.

New brain imaging techniques prove that patients with fibromyalgia experience pain from innocuous stimuli.

Scientific Research Can Help Determine the Causes of Diseases

The concept disease

Medicine is all about the study and prevention of disease. Surprisingly, though, there isn't a universally accepted definition. According to the reductionist theory, the essence of disease can be described as an ostensible injury to the body. On the contrary, holism argues that disease is caused by dysfunction. We agree with the second. Organic damage and dysfunction are not diseases. However, dysfunction, without or with organic damage is actually disease. Disease is any alteration to the body function that causes suffering.

Humankind has made many advances in understanding various diseases. These discoveries were not made randomly or by accident. It is the result a lot of hard work that has been done by many people who have followed a scientific investigation.

Scientific investigation

Philosophically speaking, scientific inquiry can be defined as the pursuit of knowledge and new ideas. For medicine, the focus of research is on finding causes for diseases and then preventing them from happening. Research has allowed for important breakthroughs in the diagnosis and treatment of many ailments. This has undoubtedly increased and prolonged the quality of human lives. One noble example is scientific research that helped eradicate polio. Although many diseases have been eradicated, there is always more to be done. The number of chronic incurable and new illnesses is constantly increasing.

Any scientific investigation, especially ones involving humans, must adhere strictly to ethical standards. Participants should be told in detail about the purpose. You should inform them about any potential risks involved in the tests that they will be performing. Their cooperation should be entirely voluntary and without coercion. To supervise and approve projects in research institutions, there must also be an ethics board.

Researchers must be creative, passionate, obsessive, and have a deep knowledge about the subject they will examine. The scientific method revolves around one central question. Let's say, what causes fibrimyalgia. A hypothesis (a tentative explanation for the central problem) is created to answer this question. Then, the method to test this hypothesis must be described in detail. A clinical study that compares a group with a disease to another group is more reliable. It is necessary to compare the drug to an inert material with a similar appearance to determine its efficacy. This will avoid false interpretations caused by unforeseeable factors such as Chapter 4, the famous placebo effect. Researchers should not determine if the results were obtained from a patient, or from a control subject to avoid bias when comparing them. The results are statistically examined to determine if the differences are real and not just random. The scientific report must then be reviewed by other investigators and then published in scientific journals.

Investigators are best to keep the process quiet and hardy. The truth is that investigation can never be perfected, but it can be confirmed.

As Schopenhauer put it:

Thus the task isn't so much to see something that no one has seen yet.

However, to think something that no one else has ever thought

>>>

Science truth is never perfect and will be challenged tomorrow. This is what makes science exciting. The future will reveal the answers to medical mysteries.

Summary

An alteration in the functioning of the body can cause pain or shorten life expectancy.

Scientific research has led to the discovery of many solutions.

The life expectancy of humans has increased.

The struggle isn't over, however. There are many diseases such as Fibromyalgia that require treatment.

Fibromyalgia in the Eyes of Many Physicians

The 20th-century's great scientific progress was in large part due to a linear, reductionist approach to the problems. Linear means the search to find a direct relationship between a phenomenon's cause and effect. Linear systems are characterized by the proportionality of the stimulus' intensity and the response's magnitude. This is how machines are made. The faster the bike goes, the more we pedal. The reductionist technique breaks down the phenomenon and breaks it down into its individual parts. Each fragment is examined individually in order to gain a better understanding of the whole. Again, we will look at machines. Watchmakers examine every part in a reductionist fashion to identify the broken gear when it breaks. The linear and reductionist paradigms imply that "the sum of all its components is equal."

In medicine, the linear approach is based in clinical-anatomical correlation. A well-defined structural cause (the cause), should match a series of symptoms and signs, or the effect. If you experience sudden, severe chest pain, along with cold sweat, it could be due to a heart attack. The cause is an obstruction in the artery that supplies blood to the heart. This reasoning states that if there are no clinical-anatomical correlates, it is likely that there isn't a disease or it falls within the scope of psychiatry. An approach that is linear cannot explain complex diseases such fibromyalgia.

The medical field is a vast one. It has been attempted to simplify medical practice into several specialties. This system of reductionism has enabled specialized physicians to have a deeper but limited view of their patients' suffering and needs. Ophthalmologists (cardiologists) and gastroenterologists are able to examine specific areas of the human anatomy in depth, but often lose their overall vision. This medical reductionism might be effective to treat linear diseases such heart attacks, hemorhoids, and cataracts. But it is cumbersome and ineffective when dealing with complex conditions such fibromyalgia. Fibromyalgia sufferers often have multiple symptoms. Because of this, they need to be seen by different specialists. Each specialist orders multiple studies to identify the source of the symptoms. This fragmentation does not provide a clear diagnosis and is a frustration for both patients as well as physicians.

The 20th century saw remarkable advances in understanding many of the linear diseases through the use of the linear-reductionist methodology. The rapid advancement of imaging techniques allowed us to see inside our bodies in detail, without the need to cut our skin. It is possible to see inside the body and determine the cause of most cancerous or infectious diseases. Microscopes are more accurate and allow us access the innermost cells. The microscope lets us see into a world that was once unseen.

Scientific knowledge is continually improving. It is now possible to see a new scientific reality, based upon the theory of chaos or complexity. This new holistic paradigm is a coherent theoretical framework which can be applied to fibromyalgia, and other complex illnesses as well.

Summary

High tech medicine offers a partial and inert understanding of diseases. It can only explain symptoms resulting from clearly defined lesions in the body.

Medical specialties artificially divise patients and their suffering.

Fibromyalgia cannot easily be understood by a simplistic and reductionist perspective.

New scientific realities are available that offer a dynamic, integrated perspective on the suffering of patients. This is an innovative way to understand complex diseases such fibromyalgia.

Fibromyalgia can be understood using new complexity sciences

Scientists saw the universe in a simple, ordered linear structure that allowed for the existence of cause and effect. The discovery that the universe was filled with random systems, despite the fact that they behave in a predictable way and there is no relation between cause and effect, has been made possible by the advent of cybernetics. These are called complex system.

A complex system is composed of multiple interwoven elements. These units interact constantly to create new properties. These systems are constantly changing to adapt to the surrounding environment. Energy flows though them. Complex adaptive system are diverse and plentiful in every realm. Complex adaptive systems can be seen in complex places like stock markets or ant colonies, democratic societies and schools, as well, as stock market, stock markets and schools, of fish. An example of a complex adaptive systems is the autonomic neural system, which we'll discuss later.

Another fascinating concept, the fractal, is a result of complexity sciences. A fractal can be described as a geometric structure with a "similarity to it." It shows the same appearance at different scales. Many organs of our bodies have fractal geometries. This is best illustrated by the lungs. Bronchi are subdivided thousands to even thousands of times. As such, the macroscopic appearances for the bronchial branch and its subdivisions can only be seen through a microscope. Fractal structures have extraordinary capacities for exchange and absorption. Their intrinsic beauty is perhaps the most convincing proof that they are true. Mandelbrot stated, "Afractals allow you to view infinity through the eyes your mind."

Fractals and complex systems cannot be understood if only their parts are studied. In this instance, linear-reductionist techniques are absolutely useless. Complexity sciences are a confirmation of the Aristotelian postulate "The whole is distinct from the sum total of its parts."

Complexity sciences are a reminder that the human being is not a machine. It is not possible to comprehend each of its parts individually. It can only be understood when you understand the interaction of its physical and mental parts with the environment. This interaction produces new properties, or "emerging", that cannot easily be explained by studying each individual component. Let's say that thought is man's greatest skill. Thought is a result of interactions among a multitude neuronal networks, yet we cannot find evidence of it or trace of it no matter how hard we probe them individually.

Complexity sciences show us that our bodies must be able to adapt to change. This is the essence of good health. This is resilience. It refers to the ability to adapt to change and give us strength. If our adaptive systems lose resilience, they will degrade and can lead to diseases such as Fibromyalgia.

This new understanding has led scientists to adopt a scientific holism approach to medical care and treatment of disease and health. This outlook suggests that the best method to deal with complex diseases such fibromyalgia would be to view each individual as a "whole", a biopsycho-social unit that is constantly adapting to its environment. This outlook recognizes that all chronic diseases have psychological repercussions. But, it is important to recognize that the environment has a profound impact on our health.

We commonly associate the term "holism" with complementary or alternative medicine. It is an esoteric concept without any scientific backing, but the theory on chaos and complexity gives holism scientific support. Orthodox medicine should recognize with humility that alternative medicine is leading the way in this matter. Holism doesn't exist as a philosophical idea, but is a new scientific reality.

Reductionism and holism do not have to be considered opposing views. They are complementary. Both visions are useful in understanding reality.

Summary

The universe is filled with complex systems that can't all be explained by looking at each part separately.

Human bodies also have flexible complex systems that adapt to constantly changing environments.

The main adaptive system that human beings have is the autonomic neurological system.

Fibromyalgia and other conditions can result from the breakdown of elasticity or resilience in complex systems.

Understanding these diseases requires holistic views, taking a holistic approach to understanding human beings; their physical alterations as well as their emotional repercussions. Also, considering the effects of the environment on health or development.
Fibromyalgia Causes

The hypothesis of fibromyalgia has to not only explain the cause of intense pain but also the reasons why someone will have different symptoms, such as fatigue or insomnia.

Predisposition genetic

Fibromyalgia is genetically predisposed. This disease is more common in patients whose immediate relatives are affected than in the general population. Twin studies have shown that roughly half of the causes for fibromyalgia can be attributed to genetic factors and half to environmental factors. As we have already mentioned, fibromyalgia sufferers can often be affected by genetic variations in an enzyme that isn't able to remove adrenaline properly from their bodies. These cases can also lead to a defect in adrenaline receptors which regulate blood pressure.

Environmental factors

Fibromyalgia could be caused by various types of infections, such as physical trauma (car accident), emotional trauma (sexual assault, death of a close relative, loss of job, divorce), and/or trauma to the brain.

Canadian researchers Moldofsky (and Smythe) conducted the first scientific studies on the development mechanisms for fibromyalgia. They showed that patients suffering from Fibromyalgia experience changes in their EEG during sleep. These anomalies result in an intrusion by alpha waves during delta wave periods, or deep sleep. Thus, sleep is unrested and fragmented.

These researchers also demonstrated that healthy subjects would develop fibromyalgia symptoms when they are subjected to repeated interruptions in deep sleep stages over several days.

The discovery of hormonal disorders was made later. Different glands produce hormones (pituitary-, thyroid-, and adrenal). Their action takes place away from the site they are produced. It has been proven that fibromyalgia results in hormonal axis modifications that produce cortisol. This substance is very similar and effective to cortisone. Cortisol is produced within the adrenal cortex. It reacts to any stress. It provides energy for the body to cope with the increased demands made by stressful stimuli.

Patients suffering from fibromyalgia were found to produce less cortisol than necessary when confronted with different stimuli. Another hormone that is incorrectly produced by patients with Fibromyalgia is the growth hormone. This hormone is most commonly produced at night by the pituitary. It is located in the center of your brain. The body's growth hormone plays a major role in adolescence. A smaller amount of growth hormone is produced by adults. This helps preserve muscle mass. One subgroup of patients with Fibromyalgia is known to have low levels of growth hormone.

EEG and hormonal studies may provide an explanation for sleep disorders and fatigue but it would not explain the main symptoms of fibromyalgia - pain.

Substance P is a primary transmitter of pain. Multiple researchers have found that people suffering from fibromyalgia have high amounts of this substance in their brain fluid. The neural growth hormone, an additional pain transmitter, was also found in them.

The new imaging methods that are used to study the brain allow us to detect subtle changes previously unnoticed. A new technology called Single Photon Emission Computed Tomography (SPECT) was used to show that patients with fibromyalgia have decreased bloodflow in certain parts of the brain. It is especially evident in the Thalamus, which is a center responsible for suppressing painful sensations and also controls the functions of the autonomic neuro system. These imaging methods show that patients suffering from Fibromyalgia activate the parts of their brain that register pain when presented with innocuous stimuli.

There have also been abnormalities in neurotransmitter expression. Nervous impulses move along nerve fibers in the same way as electrical currents. The synapses are the places where substances acting as messengers are created. These substances, which are called neurotransmitters (or messengers), allow communication among different fibers to ensure continuity of nerve impulses. Serotonin is just one such substance that has many benefits, including the ability to improve mood. Patients suffering from Fibromyalgia had lower levels of similar products to serotonin.

A significant step forward in the research on fibromyalgia pain was to realize that these patients' central pain pathways are sensitive. One possibility is that the nerves involved in pain transmission are permanently irritated. There is evidence that patients can experience the so-called windup phenomenon of pain stimuli. This phenomenon is explained in Chapter 3. It is due in part to an irregularity in the spinal chord that causes pain intensity to increase and constant perception. This is why even harmless stimuli such as grasping with moderate strength an arm can be painful.

As mediators for chronic pain, glial cells from the spinal chord have been given special attention in the last year. Long time, it was thought that these cells were a support system for the neuronal structures. Recent studies have shown that neuronal substance can be produced after significant trauma. These substances may activate glial cellular cells like Fractalkine. After being activated, glial cells produce substances called proinflammatory Cytokines which can induce pain. At the moment, it is being determined if fibromyalgia sufferers have altered glial cell functions.

Summary

Recent scientific research has allowed us to make significant progress in our understandings of fibromyalgia.

This condition is often caused by genetic predisposition.

There are well-recognized triggers like emotional trauma and infections.

Patients sleep are disturbed and do not feel refreshed.

The fluid that bathes the brains of people with Fibromyalgia contains high levels, pain-causing substances.

There is a low response of the internal cortisone system to different stimuli.

A sub-group has decreased growth hormone levels.

New imaging techniques revealed that patients had reduced blood flow in the brain thalamus. This region is responsible for pain inhibition.

They have low levels similar to serotonin.

They experience a state called "central senseization", where the nerve pathways that transmit pain to the brain are constantly irritated.

Our Progress in Understanding Fibromyalgia.

Our research group at the National Institute of Cardiology Mexico has studied the causes of fibromyalgia since many years. This is mainly through the use of forefront cardiology technologies.

Our hypothesis was, that every manifestation fibromyalgia might be explained by a modification in the autonomic nerve system. Chapter 6 provides details on the key features of this primary environmental regulation and adaptation system. The primary component of the stress reaction system is the autonomous nervous system. Although the function of the autonomic nervous system was not understood until recently, it has been transformed by the advent of sophisticated computational calculations. The heart rate variability analysis.

We used this technology for a study of 30 patients with fibromyalgia. Then we compared their results to those of 30 healthy women. All participants were recorded for 24 hours using a portable tape recording device (Holter monitor). They then went about their normal lives. Patients with fibromyalgia were found to have an incessantly overactive sympathetic nervous systems. This abnormality was particularly noticeable during sleep. In a second study, we found an association between nighttime changes in heart rate and severe fibromyalgia symptoms.

Another investigation involved another group of patients with fibromyalgia. We asked them to stand up when they had been lying down for 15 minute. The findings showed that patients with the condition did not respond to being forced to stand. Healthy people acting as a comparison group had electrocardiogram changes that indicated an immediate response from the sympathetic systems.

Our findings show that fibromyalgia has a significant alteration on the stress response system function. It is characterised by constant sympathetic activity, particularly at night. It means that there is an adrenaline excess 24 hours a week, and no normal decrease in this substance during sleep. A lack of response to stress can lead to sympathetic hyperactivity. The inability to respond to stimuli can easily be explained if you consider that a continuously accelerated system will eventually reach its limits and stop being able to respond to additional stimuli. In physiology, this is called a "ceiling phenomenon".

This type of study has been replicated elsewhere in the world by scientists who have reached similar conclusions. All of these investigations indicate that fibromyalgia may be caused by a dysfunction in the autonomic neurological system. This is due to constant hyperactivity of our sympathetic system leading us to produce excessive adrenaline. The system is unable to respond (hyporeactive), due to constant hyperactivity.

These abnormalities may explain all symptoms. Constant fatigue can be explained by a lack of response to additional stimuli. This is similar what would happen if a machine was constantly being forced to do more: it would be unable respond to any attempt of acceleration, as it is already at its maximum capacity. Fibromyalgia patients are the same. Because their regulation system has been continuously increased 24 hours a days, it is no longer capable of carrying out additional tasks. Patients feel tired and "beaten" all day.

Here's a little bit about low bloodpressure, which is common among patients suffering from fibromyalgia. Patients with high sympathetic activity would expect to have high levels of blood pressure, as adrenaline stimulates and constrains blood vessels. Yet, the opposite is true. This paradox can be explained in part by the way adrenaline hormone receptors react with chronic stimulation. It has been proven that adrenaline receptors can become desensitized by persistent stimulation. People with fibromyalgia can also be genetically deficient in adrenaline receptors. With chronic stimuli to the pain receptors, it is a different story. They become more acutely sensitive and can transmit pain even more intensely. There is sufficient scientific evidence supporting these claims.

The reason for the absence of restful sleeping is nocturnal sympathic hyperactivity. Two types were carried out simultaneously during the fibromyalgia patients' sleep. One we used heart rate variability analysis to determine how the sympathetic nervous system was functioning. On the second hand, we did polysomnography studies that not only examined the electroencephalogram but also looked at breathing patterns, body movements, as well as other variables. We compared patients who had fibromyalgia and healthy women the same year. Our previous study showed that patients with fibromyalgia have incessant, nighttime sympathetic hyperactivity. The EEG confirmed excessive startles and nighttime awakenings. It is possible that sympathetic hyperactivity may be causing these symptoms. Other study with healthy people found that EKG data of sympathetic hyperactivity precede the electroencephalographic waves that define awakening. This evidence indicates that sleep disorders such as fibromyalgia may be due to nocturnal sympathetic hypoactivity.

An adrenaline surplus can also be responsible for anxiety and nervousness. People who get an adrenaline shot feel uneasy and trembling. The same mechanism could account for cold and sometimes bluish skin.

This would explain the dryness in eyes, and mouth. It is a well-known association. Anyone who's ever been asked to speak in public knows the feeling.

Other authors have conducted heart rate variability research on patients suffering from irritable bowel syndrome. Their results are similar as ours: sympathetic hyperactivity, deficient response stress.

Research on noninfectious cystitis (the medical name is interstitial cystitis) merits further attention. This condition often coexists alongside fibromyalgia. There are signs such as urgency, burning and pain when you urinate. Cystitis symptoms are best treated by a specialist because they are well-defined in the bladder. Interstitial cystitis can lead to high levels of adrenaline. However, biopsies on the bladder wall of patients with interstitial Cystitis have shown an increase number of sympathetic nervous fibers.

Another important characteristic of interstitial cystitis that can aid in investigation of its causes is that animal models are available. This pathology can be seen in cats. In these animals, both the increased production of sympathetic fibres and an excess of adrenaline have been proven to occur.

It is possible that sympathetic hyperactivity might also be responsible in some cases of immunological changes seen in fibromyalgia. It has been demonstrated that sympathetic hyperactivity blocks Th1 response, an immune reaction that defends us from fungal infections. Alternately, sympathetic hyperactivity may increase Th2 responses, which are responsible for immunity to allergic reaction.

One mystery in fibromyalgia, however, is the cause of such disparities between genders. This is because nine women suffer from the condition for every man. Although it is not clear what the answer is, it is interesting to observe that the male sympathetic nervous system and female sympathetic nerve system are quite different in function and structure. This is more evident in animal models. Females become more interconnected with their pain pathways and sympathetic system after trauma. It is well-known that women have a higher baseline sympathetic tone than men. This can be seen as a common yet under-appreciated phenomenon. Women are more likely to have damper and colder hands than the men. This peculiarity may be caused by hormones that women have.

Another factor that contributes to constant sympathetic hyperactivity, and constant adrenaline excretion is our modern stressful environment. We live in an environment of constant misinformation. We are living a mad existence. Industrialization has caused the loss of night and day cycles. It used be that nightfall brought darkness, silence and rest. Today, you can hear light, noise, and activity at nights. Current diets are unhealthy. Exercise has been dropped. Interfamilial relationships and work environments are often difficult.

People adapt to stressful living situations by forcing their main regulation (the autonomic neuro system) to work. Sometimes, however, the system malfunctions and disease can develop. People with a genetic condition that makes them more susceptible to illness are those who don't have enough adrenaline in their system.

Summary

Advanced EKG research has shown that patients suffering from Fibromyalgia are affected by a major alteration in their stress response (the autonomic nerve system).

The system becomes less elastic due to constant day and night hyperactivity. This can lead to an excessive production of adrenaline 24 hours a week.

This alteration can explain the many manifestations of the condition.

Fibromyalgia might be thought of as a failure in the main adaptive system's attempt to adapt to an increasingly hostile world.

Chapter 6: Autonomic Nervous System

Dysfunction Also Explains Pain

The most prominent features of fibromyalgia are generalized pain and hypersensitivity, both which can be explained by changes in the functioning of the autonomic nerve system through a mechanism known sympathetically maintained pain.

We believe that fibromyalgia's pain is neuropathic. It means that the pain is caused intrinsically by a change in pain transmitting neuros. Neuropathic pain may also include long-term pain, chronic diabetes, and pain following infection with the herpeszoster virus (the post-herpes nervousgia).

Fibromyalgia resembles neuropathic pain.

* Patients do not feel any pain from ostensible damage to their joints, muscles or ligaments.

* Neuropathic pain may be accompanied, as explained in Chapter 3, by abnormal sensations (paresthesia), which can include burning, feeling tingling, cramping or discomfort when wearing tight clothes. Our

research shows that most patients suffering from Fibromyalgia experience these sensations.

* Allodynia is another characteristic of neuropathy. It is pain that is elicited by a normal painless stimulus (such touching an arm or applying pressure on the neck). We have already seen that fibromyalgia can be defined by the presence or absence of pain-palpable areas.

* Neuropathic discomfort can also be caused by central sensitization of pain pathways. This is reflected in the windup phenomena described under Chapter 3. The central sensitization of fibromyalgia has been proven to be an abnormality.

The idea of considering fibromyalgia to be a form neuropathic is being accepted by the scientific community, even though it is a new concept. This classification offers two benefits: it makes it possible for scientists to learn more about the mechanisms and treatment of neuropathy and to apply that knowledge to fibromyalgia. It also supports the validity of fibromyalgia. There is no doubt that pain can be experienced in the case trigeminal, post-herpes or other forms of neuropathy. A 2013 German study supports our assertion that fibromyalgia could be caused by neuropathy. Small fiber neuropathy, a form of neuropathic fibromyalgia, can be diagnosed using function tests on the skin's sympathetic nerves. This can also be confirmed by microscopy studies of skin biopsies. This kind of neuropathy was common in people with Fibromyalgia, according to the German study.

This subgroup is known as neuropathic, and it is caused by excessive sympathic activity. In this case, the excessive sympathetic traffic causes pain to be worsened by injecting adrenaline.

Fibromyalgia is characterized by the following sympathetic modifications

* There is ongoing sympathic hyperactivity as demonstrated by several heart rate variability studies.

* When the sympathetic systems is blocked, pain levels decrease. Scandinavian researchers have found that when fibromyalgia is blocked by an important sympathetic gland in the neck (known as the

"stellate" ganglion), there is less pain in the area within this ganglion.

* Fibromyalgia patients who have been injected with adrenaline experience increased pain. In one of our studies patients were given small amounts (placebo) and minimal amounts of adrenaline. Patients and physicians did not know the exact substance that they had been given. The same procedure also was used on patients with rheumatoidarthritis, a chronic pain disease that affects the spine, and a healthy group. The results revealed that most fibromyalgia sufferers felt pain after the adrenaline infusion, but not among the other two control group.

Neuropathic pain mediated in part by the sympathetic systems usually occurs after significant trauma. Reflex sympathetic reflex shares many commonalities with fibromyalgia. Both disorders are more common in women. They often occur after trauma. Both conditions are characterized by dysfunctions in the sympathetic nervous, which can manifest as pain, paresthesia, or hypersensitivity for palpation. Both conditions respond to sympathetic pathway blocking.

We propose that fibromyalgia can be described as a generalized version of reflex sympathetic dystrophy.

Our new research opened up to us when we discovered that fibromyalgia was a painful, neuropathic syndrome. This is due to sympathetic hyperactivity. It enabled us to apply the most recent information about the mechanisms underlying neuropathic suffering to our fibromyalgia research. Clear animal models show that neuropathic pain can be sympathetically maintained. Following trauma (physical and emotional), abnormal connections develop between the pain-conveying neurons and the sympathetic nervous system. These short-circuits happen in the dorsal Root Ganglia. It is home to a unique type of sodium channels that act like pain gatekeepers. These sodium channels have a different genetic structure in severe fibromyalgia patients than those found in healthy people. These findings suggest that in severe fibromyalgia some pain "gatekeepers' may not be working properly. These findings suggest that there are other treatment options for Fibromyalgia. This structure is well understood, and it is therefore possible to design fine analgesic medicines to specifically block them. These drugs wouldn't have the adverse effects of current medication.

Summary

The stress response system in fibromyalgia patients has changed using a new computer technique called heart rate variability assessment.

The main component to the stress response is called the autonomic neuro system.

It is characterized by persistent hyperactivity in a sympathetic (accelerator), branch, and excessive adrenaline. This causes insomnia.

This forces the system to exhaust and becomes incapable of responding appropriately to stimuli. This is what causes fatigue.

These alterations in the nervous system of the autonomic organ provide a solid explanation for other signs of fibromyalgia.

We suggest that fibromyalgia may be due to an intrinsically altered pain transmitting neuros. This phenomenon has been called neuropathic.

We think that fibromyalgia may be caused by an excessive amount of adrenaline. This is known to be sympathetically maintained or pain.

We suggest that the short circuits between sympathetic system and pain pathways are found in special nodules lying along the spinal column called "dorsalroot ganglia."

Holistic Therapy

When treating many diseases of the body, the patient acts as a recipient or a consumer of medications. Fibromyalgia requires a different approach. For fibromyalgia to be managed, both patients and their relatives must be proactive and assertive. Effective treatment starts with understanding the disease.

It isn't a real disease. That pain and other symptoms can be real. And that there is a consistent explanation for why they appear at different times.

Understanding that the nerves involved in pain perception are actually irritated does not mean that the pain is progressive in the muscles, joints and other internal structures.

Recognize that the main mechanism responsible for internal regulation of the environment and adjustment is now broken down. You may experience an emotional reaction that can cause the condition to persist.

From a philosophical perspective, fibromyalgia in many cases can be viewed as an unsuccessful adaptation to a hostile environment.

The main reasons fibromyalgia occurs in our modern world are explained below. Modernity has made our environment more hostile, as we've already stated. People try to adjust to the new world by activating their main stress response. Fibromyalgia can cause the body to lose resilience, crack and then lead to illness. To put an extreme amount of stress on our adaptive system, either emotional or physically, is detrimental.

It's important to realize that people suffering from fibromyalgia often are perfectionists and rigid. They do not feel satisfied with how they perform and often seek out the help of others.

When this is understood it is obvious that everything that leads to a happy and peaceful lifestyle is good for you. However, advice like "relax"and "keep your face up" are meaningless if they don't come with the proper tools and support.

The second component of a successful approach is to face the disease. Rehabilitation requires the participation of both the patient as well as her family. Fundamental tools for treatment are understanding and support. They shouldn't be expecting to find a cure.

Many people feel relief when they find out they have fibromyalgia. They do this because, after years, there is a clear explanation for their symptoms. Patients who have been incorrectly diagnosed and treated as if suffering from a degenerative disease will feel more relief. It is also possible to avoid having to travel all the time to get a diagnosis.

Fibromyalgia can also experience similar problems to those with chronic diseases like diabetes, hypertension and osteoarthritis. The severity spectrum starts at normal, then gradually goes up to disability. One sub-group of patients is able to go on as normal with their lives without needing an explanation. Others may need additional intervention to get on with their lives.

Each patient must receive a personalized, holistic treatment. Personalized because two patients may respond in different ways to the same treatment. You must tailor your treatment plan to meet the needs of each patient. Because every person is a biopsycho-social unit, the therapy should be holistic. The emotional and physical effects of each case must be considered. Holistic treatment can be achieved using many techniques and disciplines. It is absurd today to believe that a magic bullet will heal all fibromyalgia-related problems.

Summary

It is essential to fully understand the symptoms and treatment options.

Fibromyalgia may be described as an attempt to adapt to a hostile world.

The pain is real. However, this does NOT mean that there is any permanent damage to your muscles, bones, and joints.

Chronic pain can create negative emotional changes which need to be treated.

Patients who are fully informed should take a leadership role in their own rehabilitation in partnership with their families as well as health professionals.

There is no one-size fits all treatment. You will need to tailor the treatment to each patient.

Non-Medication Methods

A number of controlled studies have shown that certain techniques can effectively improve the symptoms fibromyalgia. It is important for us to stress that this is about improving, not curing.

Attitude towards disease

The prognosis of a patient who accepts the existence and is capable of handling the symptoms is more favorable. In contrast, patients who are devastated by the disease and unable react or take steps to improve their condition, feel helpless, depressed, or fearful, tend to be more optimistic. This is true not only for fibromyalgia. It also applies to other rheumatic disorders like osteoarthritis.

There are several techniques for psychological self-efficacy that include:

* Setting achievable goals for exercise and reaching them.

* Following others who have overcome their disease and seeing how they do it.

* Receiving positive feedback from patients, health professionals.

* Understanding the physiological reactions within the body. Realizing that adrenaline levels are constantly high can lead to numerous discomforts.

This can easily be achieved through small self-help group.

Group therapy

Group therapy for fibromyalgia with 10 to 15 patients is beneficial. For fibromyalgia to be effective, the group must possess a proactive attitude and require two key characters. The first character is a rehabilitated person who can demonstrate that there is an escape from fibromyalgia. The second character is a psychologist who is experienced in cognitive-behavioral approaches and is familiar about the disease. It is important that the group strive for improvement. Ineffective group therapies can become a whining gathering. Group therapy has the added advantage of reducing treatment expenses. It is obvious that this is not suitable for all cases of Fibromyalgia.

Exercise

Pain and fatigue are two of the most common complaints. These symptoms can be directly counterproductive to exercising. Patients may protest that it is impossible for them to exercise when they are so weak. It means that each patient should be given the right amount of exercise to suit their needs. The benefits of exercise are also supported by scientific evidence. Exercise can be used to treat fibromyalgia symptoms such as fatigue, pain, tender points, and fatigue.

We recommend starting with some stretching exercises. It is also advised to move in the water (aqua¬aerobics). Aerobic exercise includes swimming, cycling, walking and relaxing in a quiet area. Muscle strengthening exercises are suggested for advanced rehabilitation. Moving to different styles of dance is another option. Because they can disrupt your sleep, it is important to practice physical therapies in the morning.

Yin-Yang principles are the basis for many Asian disciplines such yoga, Tai Chi, and Qigong. These movements are recommended for patients with fibromyalgia because they can help improve the function of the autonomic nerve system. Tai Chi may improve the symptoms.

Breathing exercises, which directly affect the autonomic system, are very beneficial. Diaphragmatic breaths decrease adrenaline levels. Follow these steps to learn how to do this type of breathing.

* Laying down with a pillow under your knees is the starting position

* Place one side of your chest over the navel. As you breathe in (inhale), your abdomen should become larger, and your thorax should be slightly smaller.

* Keep inhaling slowly through the nose. Then exhale through slightly tightened lips. Your pace should be about 6 times per minute.

* Sessions must last no more than 5-10 seconds.

* The diaphragmatic respiration is simulated by miming a yawn.

Cognitive-behavioral therapy

The therapy consists of a series mental strategies that help patients see how different kinds of thoughts, emotions, and beliefs can affect the symptoms of their disease. A patient's role in improving their health is also highlighted. The patient is taught techniques to reduce her discomforts. One example is to make time for relaxation using meditation, breath exercises, biofeedback or image visualisation. There are also ways to restructure patients' beliefs about their disease.

It is crucial to emphasize that scientific evidence supports the benefits of the above mentioned disciplines in fibromyalgia. Although it is unclear what the cause of this improvement was, several studies have concluded that they also improve the functioning and function of the nervous system. This may be the reason that fibromyalgia symptoms have improved.

Diet

There are many patients suffering from irritable stool syndrome. It must be considered "intestinal fibromialgia" since the same conditions (painful, hypersensitive to pressure, and dysfunctional autonomic nervous systems) have been confirmed in the digestive track. Many people can see a direct connection between the intensity and distribution of intestinal discomfort.

Irritating bowel Syndrome can also be caused when the environment is hostile. In this case, it is usually due to junk food. It is difficult to find any research that examines the role diet plays in improving fibromyalgia. It is clear that there are many ways to treat the disease. You may be able to reduce certain food items and monitor the improvement over several weeks.

It's a good rule of thumb to avoid food high in animal oil, including fried foods, as they can be very spicy. You should eat mostly vegetarian diet. Red meat should be avoided.

Age slowly reduces the ability of the bowel (lactose), to absorb sugars in milk. Also, there are lactose intolerances. This is why it is important that you test the effects of avoiding fresh milk and fresh cheese.

Foods with a high amount of simple sugar (candy and pastries) should not be eaten as they can ferment and cause abdominal distention. These carbohydrates can also cause a slow decrease in glucose levels. The sudden entry of sugars in the body causes overproduction insulin and reactive hypoglycemia.

It is also advised to not drink too much alcohol or drinks that contain caffeine. Therefore, it is best to cut down on cola soft drink and coffee consumption. While this is a theory, it is possible that diet sodas may have an irritating effect on fibromyalgia patients due to their similarity to aspartate. This means that it is best to avoid drinking such beverages. Monosodium glutamamate is used in food flavoring to improve its taste. It's found in Asian foods as a condiment and in canned soups, fried food and chips.

Low blood pressure is a frequent problem for patients suffering from this disease. It can increase symptoms such as fatigue, dizziness, and dizziness. High mineral water content is an easy way to raise blood pressure. High levels of minerals in commercial sport drinks is not a good idea as they also provide glucose and other substances.

Smoking

Smoking is a serious problem. These are also the facts. Smokers have a greater chance of developing fibromyalgia. Additionally, patients suffering from fibromyalgia are more likely than non-smokers to experience discomforts.

Sleep hygiene

The lack of fresh sleep is a major problem in fibromyalgia patients. It can also lead to fatigue and increased pain. For proper circadian rhythm to function, adequate sleep is crucial. These measures can help us adjust our biological clock.

* You should get up and go to bed each day at the same time. This is a fundamental routine to regulate the biological clock. Even when your sleep quality is poor it should not be a problem to get up at the exact same hour.

* Avoid sleeping during the workday.

* No alcohol after 6 hours. While alcohol may be immediatesedative, in the long-term it can act as a stimulant.

* A light dinner is a good option, but you don't need to consume any caffeine or nicotine.

* Never exercise at night before bed.

* You should sleep in a comfortable bed.

* The bed may be used to sleep or have intimate relationships. It is not meant to be used as an office table. It should be understood that "bed" must be associated with "sleeping".

* The bedroom temperature should be kept cool. Use blankets as needed.

* Make sure you are out in the sunshine when you wake up each morning. This helps regulate our biological clock.

* Never put unfinished work or the quarrels that arose during the day to sleep.

* Establish preparative rituals. Reading, relaxing music and meditation are good choices.

* Never sleep with the TV on.

* Do Not Take Any Sleep-Altering Drugs

* If you get up in the middle night and cannot go back to bed, it is a good idea to go to another area and read something calm.

Summary

Therapy for fibromyalgia is often successful when you make important lifestyle and lifestyle changes.

There are many things you can do to alleviate the symptoms associated with fibromyalgia.

These include a positive attitude towards the condition, group therapy. Breathing exercises. Cognitive-behavioral therapy. A non-irritating vegetarian diet. No substances similar to adrenaline.

Medication as Treatment

It is important to only take medication when absolutely necessary. Self-medicating should be avoided. We've seen that fibromyalgia can cause discomfort throughout the body. The patient could end up being prescribed multiple drugs for each symptom. This includes headaches and muscle pain. The patient is at risk of side effects from taking multiple medications (polypharmacy). This can make it difficult to improve the disease. It is important to remember that people suffering from fibromyalgia tend to be very sensitive to medication. As such, it is best to start any treatment with a small dose and then gradually increase it.

The current state of medicine has made polypharmacy a perilous problem. It is because the medical profession has become fragmented and divided into different specialties. Therefore, it is best for one doctor to coordinate the treatment. He may consult with a specialist if necessary.

People often wonder what kind of specialist would be best to treat their fibromyalgia. The history of fibromyalgia is that it was first defined by rheumatologists, who then researched the disease to better understand the mechanisms. But, the current evidence proves that fibromyalgia actually is a neurological illness. We believe that rather than a well-defined doctor, the best physician for fibromyalgia is one who understands the disease and can distinguish between the many symptoms it can cause.

Pain medication

Fibromyalgia can be treated with anti-inflammatory drugs. These include celecoxib, diclofenac and naproxen. They are only used when there is an additional painful component such as osteoarthritis.

Analgesics

Pure analgesics, such as paracetamol, are more effective at initial doses of 500mg three times daily. These can be increased up to 750mg four times daily.

Tramadol has a stronger analgesic. One 50 mg tablet, three to four times daily is the recommended starting dose. This substance also comes in drops with a concentration of 10mg per milliliter. This allows the user to use a more cautious dosage. To be safe, you should only take 5-10 drops 3-4 times per day. Side effects that Tramadol can cause include nausea, dizziness, and vomiting.

When intense pain is felt, both tramadol and paracetamol can be combined.

Anti-neuropathic medication

As we have already stated, fibromyalgia also has neuropathic characteristics. There are substances you can take to decrease the pain transmission nerve's excitability. These substances are known by the name anti-neuropathic drug. They can be used for conditions like diabetic or post-herpetic nervous system disorders. But they are also effective in fibromyalgia. Gabapentin or pregabalin belong to this class. Gabapentin is recommended to take between 1200-2400 mg each day. Numerous studies have proved that pregabalin works well for fibromyalgia. It was actually the FDA's first official approval for this condition. Pregabalin may also be helpful in anxiety and insomnia. The recommendation by the pharmaceutical company is to take between 300 and 450mg daily. These drugs can cause dizziness and lethargy, which are two of the most common side reactions. Weight gain is a lesser-known adverse effect. It is important that we stress the fact that people with Fibromyalgia are sensitive to medication. According to our experience, they do not tolerate the high dosages prescribed by pharmaceutical companies. We recommend that you start with low doses of medication at night.

These compounds might be more beneficial in cases of intense pain that is accompanied by significant paresthesia (burning sensations/tingling and electric shock). An additional argument to support the neuropathic cause of fibromyalgia pain in fibromyalgia, is the fact that these anti-neuropathic compounds work in this condition.

Antidepressants

The use of antidepressants has been common in the treatment of fibromyalgia as well as other chronic pain disorders. Amitriptyline which belongs to the tricyclic antidepressant group is the most well-known. The recommended doses for treating fibromyalgia should be lower than those prescribed for depression. The first dose of amitriptyline is 10 mg at night. It can be slowly increased, but it's effective against pain, fatigue, insomnia and fatigue. Some patients experience opposite side effects, such as nocturnal anxiety, dizziness, and dry mouth during daylight hours.

Cyclobenzaprine, too, is part of the medication class with a tricyclic structure. Although it may be similar to Amitriptyline, it seems to have less antidepressant effect and a higher muscle relaxing capability. A number of controlled studies with patients with fibromyalgia show that cyclobenzaprine can have a positive influence on pain, sleep quality, tender points, and other aspects. The initial dose of 10 mg was used at night. It can be increased to up to 30 mg. These side effects are most common. A recent study revealed that cyclobenzaprine with lower dosages (between 1-2 and 4 mg at bedtime) has less side effects.

One type of antidepressant, apart from paroxetine (fluoxetine), is selective serotonin regulatory inhibitors. Patients suffering from fibromyalgia were subject to controlled trials that showed improvement in their pain and mood.

The "dual inhibitors of serotonin, adrenaline, and reuptake" antidepressants are now available. These two drugs have been proven in controlled clinical trials to significantly improve symptoms of fibromyalgia. Duloxetine should be taken in daily dosages of 60-60 mg. Start taking 30 mg each morning. These side effects include anxiety, dizziness or insomnia. Milnacipran also belongs to the same class and has a similar therapeutic approach. The daily recommended dose for fibromyalgia is between 200 and 100 mg. 50 mg daily is the recommended initial dose.

These types of medication are effective in fibromyalgia. That would be contrary to our suggestion that fibromyalgia might be an adrenaline dependent, painful syndrome. These drugs increase adrenaline accessibility. It is important to note that duloxetine inhibits sodium channels in your dorsal root-ganglia. Perhaps this is where it finds its analgesic power.

Opioids:

Fibromyalgia shouldn't be treated with strong opioids (oxycodone and morphine). Patients suffering from fibromyalgia may have reduced cerebral opioid receptors. This makes these drugs less effective. Contrary to popular belief, this medication can worsen preexisting symptoms. Opioid use has a reputation for causing constipation. Other side effects include sedation or mental clouding.

Treatments and medications under evaluation

At the moment, research is underway to determine the safety and effectiveness of various compounds. It's encouraging to see how big pharmaceutical companies finally pay attention to the study fibromyalgia. Cannabinoids, sodium oxybate and cannabinoids are just a few of the new drugs. Also, transcranial electromagnetic stimulation (TMS) is mentioned.

Cannabinoids (now under evaluation for Fibromyalgia) are analgesic substances that are derived primarily from marihuana. In the initial study, nabilone showed a slight but significant improvement in pain and sleep for patients with Fibromyalgia. Undesirable side effects include lethargy as well as nausea.

Naropepsy treatment is possible with sodium oxybate. Although the benefits of sodium oxybate were demonstrated in controlled studies, they have not been approved for this condition. It is also illegally used as a "recreational drug".

Transcranial electromagnetic stimulation is non-invasive and aims to modify the brain cortex areas that perceive pain by magnetic stimulation. There are many types and results of magnetic stimulation.

Patients are frequently afraid of the risks of becoming dependent on medication. Both of these situations must be distinguished. The patient will want to keep taking the medication because of the positive effect it has on their pain. This is not addiction. Instead, it's a dependency on the treatment's positive effects. True addiction, however, is a completely different situation. It is the illegal or dishonest use of medication to achieve euphoric effects.

An injection of xylocaine is appropriate for local pain relief in an area of the body that is especially painful.

If there is extreme pain, it's okay to inject xylocaine intravenously. While there are anecdotal evidence of positive results in medical literature it is worth noting that intravenous doses of xylocaine have the potential for serious complications.

Substances that might improve sleep

All mammals secrete a hormone to help them fall asleep when it's nightfall. It's called melatonin. It is secreted by their pineal gland. Melatonin naturally enhances sleep. Initial doses up to 3 mg can be increased by the pineal gland. This compound is also useful against transatlantic flight jet lag.

The mildly effective treatment for insomnia is the valerian root extract (Valerianaofficinalis).

One class of drugs is used for allergic reactions. Sedation is often a side effect. It is commonly used to alleviate sleeplessness. Diphenhydramine, a compound that can be taken at night (50mg), is the best.

Many doctors recommend that patients suffering from insomnia take low amounts of tricyclic depression medications such as amitriptyline. The recommended starting dose is 10 mg at night. You can also use benzodiazepine tranquilizers for this purpose. For example, clonazepam is recommended at a maximum dose of 0.25 mg each night. This compound can also serve as an anti-anxiety drug during the day. Zolpidem and Lorazepam are also included in this group.

As fibromyalgia can be accompanied by restless leg syndrome, it is often referred to as a "night companion". Iron deficiency may be one reason. The symptoms of these cases improve when iron intake is increased. Pramipexole works well in restless legs syndrome cases where iron levels have not been elevated.

It is important that all drug use be done under strict medical supervision.

Medication for irritable intestinal syndrome

Fibromyalgia is often accompanied by Irritable Bowel Syndrome. It causes severe abdominal pain, distension, and constipation. Looperamide is a drug that decreases intestinal motility. This is helpful when bowel irritation is manifested as diarrhea. These should be administered immediately without waiting for the symptoms to develop, in low doses of one tablet per day. This helps patients live a more normal and relaxed life, away from their homes, in many cases.

Local action can be used when the problem is primarily constipation. Also, sennosides and other plant substances can improve intestinal motility. Other laxatives can be used if these measures fail to suffice, such as bisacodyl and sodium picosulphate.

Agents to block adrenaline

Fibromyalgia has a high level of adrenaline production. This makes it logical to treat it by using adrenaline antagonists. Propranolol is effective in relieving pain in the temporomandibular disease. We used low doses (often 10 mg twice daily) of propranolol as an adrenaline beta blocker. We administered it to young women with fibromyalgia who had fainting, heart palpitations and anxiety crisis.

Studies are required to test whether adrenaline beta blockers reduce the pain of fibromyalgia.

Other substances also affect nerve junctions (synapses), of the brain, by modulating the neurotransmitter release from the adrenaline section. This group of neurotransmitters are also known generically as catecholamines. Tizanidine (used as a muscle relaxer) also falls within this group.

Which type of medication is best?

Different patients have different responses to medication. It is impossible to predict what will happen. To find out if compounds are useful, patients should test them. Based on the pain symptom profile, however, you can draw certain guidelines. Tricyclics agents (amitriptyline, ciclobenzaprine) can be helpful in treating sleep disorders. Pregabalin, gabapentin, which are anti-neuropathic agents, can improve sleep and reduce cramps. For those suffering from severe anxiety and depression, antidepressants (fluoxetine), paroxetine or duloxetine (or milnacipran) may be preferred.

Experts propose a combination of pharmacological treatments, as the different actions of the drugs have been mentioned. Studies have not yet been done to support this kind.

Evolution of the disease

Fibromyalgia experiences periods of exacerbation as well as periods of remission. Fibromyalgia is not an illness that gets worse with age. A Canadian three-year observation revealed that there was an improvement in the overall condition. In fact, it showed that at least 30% of patients experienced significant improvement. The cause of the improvement could not be identified.

It is apparent that there must be more effective and refined medication for fibromyalgia pain.

Chapter 7: Fibromyalgia - Prepaid Systems,

Public Health Systems. Work Disability

We've already seen the challenges in diagnosing and treating Fibromyalgia. Overcrowded health systems can make matters even worse. Even though public systems of health are different in each country, they share many common problems. One example is the overcrowding. Physicians don't have much time to see patients. The people waiting in the waiting rooms will suffer if they are given more time. Fibromyalgia causes many symptoms. It can take time and effort to determine the cause. This combination of overcrowding with a lack of time is a recipe for frustration for both the patient AND the doctor.

The fact that many doctors hesitate to treat patients with Fibromyalgia is a matter of grave concern. They are often unable to take the time to care for their multiple symptoms, lack of knowledge about the mechanisms, and have poor responses to medications. One of the greatest inefficiencies within the public health system is the lack of attention given to complex, frequent conditions like fibromyalgia.

We are 100% convinced that this condition, as well as others, should be handled in specialist clinics. It is the responsibility of physicians to diagnose the disease and then, if necessary start the appropriate medication. Once the patient's diagnosis is made, she should then be referred to a holistic program. She could be offered a range of therapeutic modalities including explanations, diet, physical therapy, psychological interventions, as well as all of the methods described in the previous chapters. Doctors will be available to answer questions. This type of program would lower waiting lists, be more efficient, and likely cost less. Do not continue to use old methods. This will only lead to frustration and discord.

A second important issue to be considered is the connection between fibromyalgia, work, and family. These symptoms can cause problems in the workplace and affect routine activities. As stated before, there are many different levels of severity for discomforts. There are people who can, after they discover the root cause of their discomforts and get on with their daily lives, live almost as normal.

On the other side, some people feel so severely affected that they cannot perform on the job. They seek financial compensation.

Both patients and doctors should aim to improve the symptoms, not seek work disability rulings. They are not the cure, but an acceptable alternative. Patients will continue to experience the symptoms of Fibromyalgia. Sometimes, work disability proceedings can place patients in a very difficult position. Patients want to improve their symptoms. However, the authorities expect them to prove their seriousness.

The trials for disability are particularly difficult when it comes to chronic pain. Because there is no objective measure of how severe the disease is, the trial will not be successful. It will always feel subjectively and privately, and be accompanied by a negative emotion. As we have already mentioned, patients with fibromyalgia don't need to be examined physically. The lab results are usually normal. There is no formula for determining who is eligible for disability.

The Nordic countries are well-known for their research that shows there is an identifiable group of patients who, regardless of their underlying condition, cannot work. These are their characteristics: they are often single, have less education and make lower incomes from work. They also tend to be older and do repetitive physical maneuvers in the workplace.

North American experts in labor medicine recommend that an integrated multidisciplinary evaluation be conducted to assess the possibility of a work disability. This includes participation by psychologists, physicians and occupational therapy professionals. It is essential to establish the existence of many factors in this assessment.

* Stress factors in the workplace that could possibly be reduced.

* Inconsistencies in work demands and patient ability to meet them.

* Determine if the person who can't bear the workload has depression, or another mental disorder that could be treated.

* Define whether the person could benefit by being granted a temporary handicap.

* Research the possibility of retraining a patient for a different type of work.

Patients suffering from Fibromyalgia enjoy the same right to work disability as those with other chronic diseases. Disability trials should include lawyers responsible for legal aspects as well as doctors who specialize in the treatment of psychological and labor conditions. You should first acknowledge the fact that fibromyalgia symptoms may be the same as any other rheumatic illness. Next, choose the best option. Rehabilitating patient health is the priority. The work environment should be matched with the individual's abilities.

Summary

Overcrowding health services make it impossible to treat patients suffering from complex diseases, such as fibromyalgia.

Look for creative alternatives. Group therapy is just one option.

Fibromyalgia is a condition that makes it difficult to do the job.

Labor disability trials must begin with the recognition that the symptoms being referred by patients are real.

There are some options for labor disabilities that can be matched to the limitations of the patient by making adjustments to the workplace environment.

Complementary Treatments and Alternatives

Complementary and alternative medicine can be described as a set of procedures or other substances from outside the scope of scientific medicine. They may help with patient discomforts but their efficacy must still be established by controlled studies.

It is important to distinguish between complementary and alternative treatments from quackery. This will be covered in the next section. As useful and potentially helpful measures in fibromyalgia treatments, complementary or alternative treatments need to be given respect.

There are many complementary medicines. These are the most well-known and applicable to fibromyalgia. It should be noted whether they have received preliminary

163

controlled trials proving their efficacy. The disadvantages and advantages of these types treatments are also briefly evaluated.

Chiropractic

Daniel David Palmer established this discipline in 1895. It is a method of relieving pain by manipulating your spine to correct vertebral underluxations. They have been trained as chiropractors and are members in good standing of the college supervision bodies. This is the main country that this treatment method originated. Chiropractic manipulations have been shown to be effective in relieving lower back pain. There is no scientific evidence to support the effectiveness of chiropractic manipulations in treating fibromyalgia.

Acupuncture

This is an ancient Chinese discipline that dates back centuries. It is based the idea of a vital force running through the body that influences its functions. Energy flows freely and harmoniously in the body. It is free from any obstructions. Again, we return to the Chapter 5 concept of ying/yang. It has been demonstrated that acupuncture elevates the levels of endorphins in our bodies, which are natural analgesics.

Acupuncture stimulates particular points in your body. Many of these points are located in the meridians. According to this philosophy, they are energy-conductive channels. It is interesting to observe the relationship between the anatomy of the meridians as well as the location for the sympathetic nervous systems ganglia. The fact that it relieves nausea in chemotherapy patients is evidence of the effectiveness of acupuncture. It is also a well-known analgesic. In fibromyalgia patients, acupuncture has been shown to reduce pain in some cases.

Homeopathy

Samuel Hahnemann, an 18-year-old scientist, created this discipline. According to him, similar cures like is a theory that substances that adversely affect a healthy individual may also be beneficial for a sick patient if the dosage is low. One method of treating a patient is to give them diluted plants. A North American research group found that patients suffering from fibromyalgia experienced more pain relief when they used verum LM (a homeopathic compound) in a controlled trial.

Natural neutraceutical supplements

These include a number of vitamins and minerals, neurotransmitters, animal product like shark cartilage, as well other natural substances, such as chondroitin, glucosamine, and S-adenosylmethionine.

A specific form of arthritis could be affected by chondroitin or glucosamine, which is known as osteoarthritis. There is no reason for them to be able to improve the symptoms fibromyalgia.

SAM-e (S-adenosylmethionine) is an interesting compound. It is created by combining L.metionine with adenosinetriphosphate. (ATP). It can interfere with various metabolic processes. It has analgesic or antidepressant properties. SAM-e proved to be more efficacious than a placebo in treating fibromyalgia. A double-blind Danish study found that 800mg of SAM e daily was more effective than a placebo. SAM–e has also been prescribed for cases of depression.

There are many natural products available that have been used in the treatment of fibromyalgia. However, these products have not been directly proven to work on the conditions.

St. John's Wort is a natural remedy for mild depression, fatigue and other symptoms. Magnesium molate may possess analgesic properties. Ginkgo biloba has been said to improve memory. However it acts in a similar way as caffeine which can make you anxious.

Coenzyme Q10 (anti-oxidant) enhances mitochondrion effectiveness. Mitochondria produce energy for cells. A severe shortage of coenzymeQ10 may cause fatigue or aches. A skin biopsy of patients with fibromyalgia revealed a reduction in the levels of this vitamin. It is unknown if this deficiency causes or effects the condition. A recent, small controlled study found that coenzymeQ10 may help with fibromyalgia.

Vitamin D deficiency is possible to cause fibromyalgia. But, it only occurs when blood levels are less than 10 nanograms/milliliter.

Vitamin D, coenzyme Q 10, and vitamin Q10 share a similar past in medicine. While both have been recommended for the treatment of multiple conditions, such as fibromyalgia or other issues, their effectiveness has been limited to a small number of diseases. Coenzyme Q10 has been shown to be useful in the treatment of rare muscular diseases called mitochondrialmyopathies. Vitamin D is useful in the treatment of osteomalacia as well as for certain calcium and/or phosphorous metabolic diseases. Although they are virtually free from undesirable effects, more research is required to verify their effectiveness.

Other types

Tai Chi is an ancient Chinese discipline. It originated in martial arts. It involves rhythmic movements combined with breathing exercises and meditation. Research is showing Tai Chi has a positive effect on fibromyalgia symptoms. Because of this, orthodox medicine is starting to accept it as part of their therapeutic regimen. Controlled studies also support the effectiveness and safety of yoga.

Balneotherapy. The evidence is clear that fibromyalgia can be improved by a variety of water therapies, including thermal baths.

Although massage can be relieving for many patients, there are many other techniques that may provide relief.

In certain situations, Hypnosis is effective. Magnets however have not proved to be efficient.

The darker side of complementary and other medicine's attraction

A lot of people feel drawn to this type of treatment because of the intrinsic value. The shortcomings of orthodox medical care, such as patronizing attitudes and lack of time given to patients or side effects and adverse effects, are some of the reasons. On the other side, society is placing greater demands on the quality of its productive lives.

It is clear that complementary therapies can also have dark side effects and be risky. Chapter 4 shows that improvement does not come from the active ingredients of the substances used but rather from the placebo effect they induce. For complementary medicine, the rigid supervision that is required for orthodox medicine cannot be applied. As a result, there are many fraudsters who claim they are doctors.

It is well known, however that complementary treatments have limited and only beneficial effects for certain types of painful conditions. Yet, many people mistakenly believe that complementary treatments are the panacea. They can treat all kinds of illnesses.

Natural products don't have to be subjected to rigorous quality control. The purity of natural products cannot be trusted. An American study revealed that 12% sold as ginseng preparations did not contain any. Furthermore, the batches that did contain some varied greatly in their ginseng levels and did NOT reflect the information on the package label.

A second problem with complementary medicine is that there are no rigorous studies to prove its effectiveness. A commitment to a particular treatment is more emotional than rational.

In many different alternative treatments, there is a constant return to the past. This is evident in homeopathy as well as chiropractic and acupuncture. Many of the principles and treatments used in these alternative therapies are very similar to those developed centuries ago. There is no single cure or science for all diseases. The solution lies in the progression of knowledge, not in the nostalgia-driven practice of ancient therapeutic rituals.

Summary

For fibromyalgia treatment, alternative methods or supplements should be considered.

There are many useful supplements, including SAMe, coenzymeQ10 vitamin D, St. John's Wort or magnesium maleate.

Yoga, Tai Chi, as well as balneotherapy, have all been proven to be efficient.

Complementary treatments can be dangerous. People who call themselves doctors, and the remedies they advocate, are not properly supervised.

The quack

The quack, a charismatic but sinister personality who has been around disease throughout the history and present-day medicine, is often portrayed as a charismatic but evil character. A quack can be described as someone who brags about being able to find a cure (generally for every chronic condition). It is quite interesting to note that, in many cases, the quack doesn't appear to be a recalcitrant lieur, but instead a person who lacks critical judgment and is unaware of the immense complexity of chronic illnesses. Sometimes, the quack can be a sociopath. He might seem seductive, charming, and conveying assurance through his statements. But he may not care about his limitations as an therapist or how he deceives the most vulnerable people in society, the chronically-ill.

The quack's profile is sufficiently distinct to be easily identified, regardless of whether it claims he can cure cancer, arthritis, or fibromyalgia. These individuals are generally not qualified to work in the field of the disease, and they may not even be doctors. They "discover" the disease by themselves, often without any support from science. Their pseudo arguments are filled with medical jargon, but cannot withstand even elementary scientific scrutiny.

They don't just want to make a contribution to the knowledge of a specific disease. They are determined to find the cure or the entire solution to all complicated diseases. They do not realize that knowledge can only be achieved through a systematic progression of ideas. It is not possible to start building from ground level without first laying a foundation.

Sometimes, their breakthrough is triggered by an accident. The evidence that it can cure (or improve) a condition is not based upon controlled studies. Instead, the evidence is always anecdotal. so and so was dying from cancer. He was completely cured after he had received my treatment. Mr. so could still exist, but he has very likely never been diagnosed with the same terminal illness. A personal testimony is one of the most common hooks to catch victims. When quacks were asked where one could find the legions

173

that they have cured with their amazing method, the answer was: Patients are so happy not to know about their diseased past.

Quacks can go beyond the limits. Quacks are able to raving about their miraculous potion, which not only heals fibromyalgia and osteoarthritis (both very different diseases), but it also works well with any form of rheumatism.

The placebo effect is their greatest ally, and Quacks who "cure rheumatic illnesses" don't even know it exists. They do not realize the fact that an analgesic should be effective if it provides relief to more people than 30%. (See Chapter 4).

A quack loves Goliath's story about David. He claims that his wondrous discovery has not been widely applied due to the economic interests of the pharmaceutical industry that conspire against it. He claims that releasing his discovery would cause them to lose their money, yet he does not fear losing his income by selling his magic product.

These quacks end up in the same place as the tragic cabaret sopranos. They have their moment, but they are soon forgotten and replaced by another person with better tricks or more seductive ways. It must be difficult for quacks to suffer from a chronic illness and live with it, knowing that he has made others vulnerable.

Quacky has attracted patients for many reasons. It is the despair that patients feel about their poor health and drives them to find any means of improving it. In order to believe in a simple solution without any reasonable support, there must be a certain level of naivety. A certain amount of irresponsibility lies behind this naivety. It is easier than to blindly believe that a miraculous product will cure your condition.

The peculiar social cultural traditions that underlie this attraction are rooted in the human desire to be rational. Magical explanations of the world and its events have been attractive to some societies for centuries. A small group of people find quackery attractive because they are opposed to the establishment. They will reject authority, orthodox medicines, the pharmaceutical industry, or government health agencies.

We are all victims of the mass dissemination of quackery by mass communications in this global village. Advertising miracle cures and other remedies for various diseases is just one example.

Information is the best tool against quackery. Information is the best resource against quackery. A knowledgeable person will review any supposedly wonderful treatments and ask about the theoretical foundation that underpins them, as well as the mechanism for their implementation and the scientific studies that back it up.

As we have already stated, fibromyalgia also has neuropathic characteristics. There are substances you can take to decrease the pain transmission nerve's excitability. These substances are known by the name anti-neuropathic drug. They can be used for conditions like diabetic or post-herpetic nervous system disorders. But they are also effective in fibromyalgia. Gabapentin or pregabalin belong to this class. Gabapentin is recommended to take between 1200-2400 mg each day. Numerous studies have proved that pregabalin works well for fibromyalgia. It was actually the FDA's first official approval for this condition. Pregabalin may also be helpful in anxiety and insomnia. The recommendation by the pharmaceutical company is to take between 300 and 450mg daily. These drugs can cause dizziness and lethargy, which are two of the most common side reactions. Weight gain is a lesser-known adverse effect. It is important that we stress the fact that people with Fibromyalgia are sensitive to medication. According to our experience, they do not tolerate the high dosages prescribed by pharmaceutical companies. We recommend that you start with low doses of medication at night.

These compounds might be more beneficial in cases of intense pain that is accompanied by significant paresthesia (burning sensations/tingling and electric shock). An additional argument to support the neuropathic cause of fibromyalgia pain in fibromyalgia, is the fact that these anti-neuropathic compounds work in this condition.

Antidepressants

The use of antidepressants has been common in the treatment of fibromyalgia as well as other chronic pain disorders. Amitriptyline which belongs to the tricyclic antidepressant group is the most well-known. The recommended doses for treating fibromyalgia should be lower than those prescribed for depression. The first dose of amitriptyline is 10 mg at night. It can be slowly increased, but it's effective against pain, fatigue, insomnia and fatigue. Some patients experience opposite side effects, such as nocturnal anxiety, dizziness, and dry mouth during daylight hours.

Cyclobenzaprine, too, is part of the medication class with a tricyclic structure. Although it may be similar to Amitriptyline, it seems to have less antidepressant effect and a higher muscle relaxing capability. A number of controlled studies with patients with fibromyalgia show that cyclobenzaprine can have a positive influence on pain, sleep quality, tender points, and other aspects. The initial dose of 10 mg was used at night. It can be increased to up to 30 mg. These side effects are most common. A recent study revealed that cyclobenzaprine with lower dosages (between 1-2 and 4 mg at bedtime) has less side effects.

One type of antidepressant, apart from paroxetine (fluoxetine), is selective serotonin regulatory inhibitors. Patients suffering from fibromyalgia were subject to controlled trials that showed improvement in their pain and mood.

The "dual inhibitors of serotonin, adrenaline, and reuptake" antidepressants are now available. These two drugs have been proven in controlled clinical trials to significantly improve symptoms of fibromyalgia. Duloxetine should be taken in daily dosages of 60-60 mg. Start taking 30 mg each morning. These side effects include anxiety, dizziness or insomnia. Milnacipran also belongs to the same class and has a similar therapeutic approach. The daily recommended dose for fibromyalgia is between 200 and 100 mg. 50 mg daily is the recommended initial dose.

These types of medication are effective in fibromyalgia. That would be contrary to our suggestion that fibromyalgia might be an adrenaline dependent, painful syndrome. These drugs increase adrenaline accessibility.

It is important to note that duloxetine inhibits sodium channels in your dorsal root-ganglia. Perhaps this is where it finds its analgesic power.

Opioids:

Fibromyalgia shouldn't be treated with strong opioids (oxycodone and morphine). Patients suffering from fibromyalgia may have reduced cerebral opioid receptors. This makes these drugs less effective. Contrary to popular belief, this medication can worsen preexisting symptoms. Opioid use has a reputation for causing constipation. Other side effects include sedation or mental clouding.

Treatments and medications under evaluation

At the moment, research is underway to determine the safety and effectiveness of various compounds. It's encouraging to see how big pharmaceutical companies finally pay attention to the study fibromyalgia. Cannabinoids, sodium oxybate and cannabinoids are just a few of the new drugs. Also, transcranial electromagnetic stimulation (TMS) is mentioned.

Cannabinoids (now under evaluation for Fibromyalgia) are analgesic substances that are derived primarily from marihuana. In the initial study, nabilone showed a slight but significant improvement in pain and sleep for patients with Fibromyalgia. Undesirable side effects include lethargy as well as nausea.

Naropepsy treatment is possible with sodium oxybate. Although the benefits of sodium oxybate were demonstrated in controlled studies, they have not been approved for this condition. It is also illegally used as a "recreational drug".

Transcranial electromagnetic stimulation is non-invasive and aims to modify the brain cortex areas that perceive pain by magnetic stimulation. There are many types and results of magnetic stimulation.

Patients are frequently afraid of the risks of becoming dependent on medication. Both of these situations must be distinguished. The patient will want to keep taking the medication because of the positive effect it has on their pain. This is not addiction. Instead, it's a dependency on the treatment's positive effects. True addiction, however, is a completely different situation. It is the illegal or dishonest use of medication to achieve euphoric effects.

An injection of xylocaine is appropriate for local pain relief in an area of the body that is especially painful.

If there is extreme pain, it's okay to inject xylocaine intravenously. While there are anecdotal evidence of positive results in medical literature it is worth noting that intravenous doses of xylocaine have the potential for serious complications.

Substances that might improve sleep

All mammals secrete a hormone to help them fall asleep when it's nightfall. It's called melatonin. It is secreted by their pineal gland. Melatonin naturally enhances sleep. Initial doses up to 3 mg can be increased by the pineal gland. This compound is also useful against transatlantic flight jet lag.

The mildly effective treatment for insomnia is the valerian root extract (Valerianaofficinalis).

One class of drugs is used for allergic reactions. Sedation is often a side effect. It is commonly used to alleviate sleeplessness. Diphenhydramine, a compound that can be taken at night (50mg), is the best.

Many doctors recommend that patients suffering from insomnia take low amounts of tricyclic depression medications such as amitriptyline. The recommended starting dose is 10 mg at night. You can also use benzodiazepine tranquilizers for this purpose. For example, clonazepam is recommended at a maximum dose of 0.25 mg each night. This compound can also serve as an anti-anxiety drug during the day. Zolpidem and Lorazepam are also included in this group.

As fibromyalgia can be accompanied by restless leg syndrome, it is often referred to as a "night companion". Iron deficiency may be one reason. The symptoms of these cases improve when iron intake is increased. Pramipexole works well in restless legs syndrome cases where iron levels have not been elevated.

It is important that all drug use be done under strict medical supervision.

Medication for irritable intestinal syndrome

Fibromyalgia is often accompanied by Irritable Bowel Syndrome. It causes severe abdominal pain, distension, and constipation. Looperamide is a drug that decreases intestinal motility. This is helpful when bowel irritation is manifested as diarrhea. These should be administered immediately without waiting for the symptoms to develop, in low doses of one tablet per day. This helps patients live a more normal and relaxed life, away from their homes, in many cases.

Local action can be used when the problem is primarily constipation. Also, sennosides and other plant substances can improve intestinal motility. Other laxatives can be used if these measures fail to suffice, such as bisacodyl and sodium picosulphate.

www.ingramcontent.com/pod-product-compliance
Lightning Source LLC
Chambersburg PA
CBHW062140020426
42335CB00013B/1276